UNDERSTANDING

DIABETES & ENDOCRINOLOGY

a problem-orientated approach

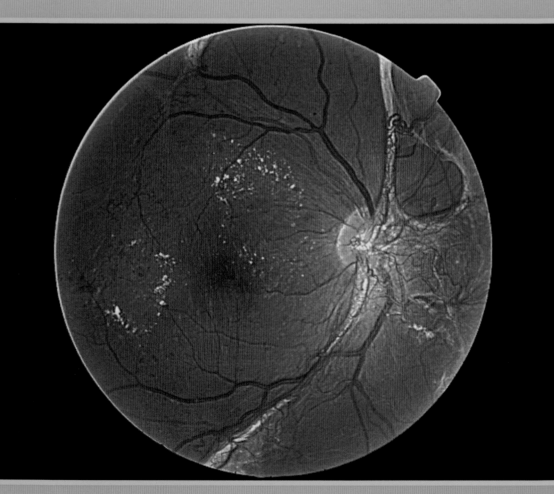

DARRYL R. MEEKING

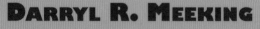

Understanding
DIABETES &
ENDOCRINOLOGY
a problem-orientated approach

Darryl R. Meeking

MBChB, MRCP
Diabetes Centre, Queen Alexandra Hospital, Portsmouth, UK

MANSON
PUBLISHING

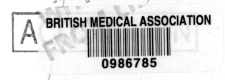

Dedication

To Penny and Daisy.

Acknowledgments

Particular thanks to Sharon Tuck and Jane Cansfield for providing the excellent photographs used in this book.

Thanks also to Dr Julia Thomas, Specialist Registrar in Endocrinology and the Departments of Endocrinology and Medical Imaging, Nuclear Medicine, and Radiology, St Bartholomew's Hospital, London for providing additional images.

For full details of all Manson Publishing Ltd titles please write to:
Manson Publishing Ltd, 73 Corringham Road, London NW11 7DL, UK.

Tel: +44(0)20 8905 5150
Fax: +44(0)20 8201 9233
Website: www.mansonpublishing.com

Commissioning editor: Jill Northcott
Project manager and copy-editor: Ruth Maxwell
Cover design: Cathy Martin, Presspack Computing Ltd
Book design and layout: Cathy Martin, Presspack Computing Ltd
Colour reproduction: Tenon & Polert Colour Scanning Ltd, Hong Kong
Printed by: Replika Press Pvt Ltd, Haryana, India

Contents

Introduction

This book aims to give the reader an understanding of the backgound, diagnosis, investigation, and management of diabetes and endocrine disease. It deliberately focuses upon diabetes, a frighteningly common and debilitating condition encountered by all doctors, regardless of specialist interest. Endocrine disease is principally a problem of glands and the abnormal quantities of hormones that they produce. Thus, for the most part, the endocrine sections of the book are set out according to the affected gland and the quantity of hormone being produced. The book also seeks to navigate the reader around the complexities of hormonal disease in a simple fashion.

This book is set out in three main sections. The first gives a background understanding of diabetes and a review of glandular systems. The second outlines the disease problems and their investigation, including the specific complications of diabetes. The third covers the management and treatment of diabetes and endocrine disease, importantly including prevention and screening.

I hope that it is an enjoyable and useful read.

Darryl R Meeking

Abbreviations

5-HIAA 5-hydroxyindole acetic acid
17-OHP 17-hydroxyprogesterone
ACE angiotensin-converting enzyme
ACR albumin:creatinine ratio
ACTH adrenocorticotrophic hormone
ADH antidiuretic hormone
AGE advanced glycation end product
ALT alanine aminotransferase
ATP adenosine triphosphate
BMI body mass index
CAH congenital adrenal hyperplasia
CAPD chronic ambulatory peritoneal dialysis
CK creatinine kinase
CLL chronic lymphocytic leukaemia
CMV cytomegalovirus
CNS central nervous system
CRH corticotrophin releasing hormone
CSF cerebrospinal fluid
CSII continuous subcutaneous insulin infusion
CT computing tomography
CVP central venous pressure
DCCT Diabetes Control and Complications Trial

DDAVP desmopressin
DEXA dual X-ray absorptiometry
DHEA dihydroepiandrostenedione
DI diabetes insipidus
DIDMOAD diabetes insipidus, diabetes mellitus, optic atrophy, and deafness
DIGAMI Diabetes Insulin Glucose Infusion in Acute Myocardial Infarction (Study)
DKA diabetic ketoacidosis
DNA deoxyribonucleic acid
DPP-IV dipeptidyl peptidase IV
DVLA Driver and Vehicle Licensing Authority
ECG echocardiogram
ED erectile dysfunction
ESR erythrocyte sedimentation rate
FH familial hypercholesterolaemia
FHH familial hypocalciuric hypercalcaemia
FNA fine-needle aspiration
FPG fasting plasma glucose
FSH follicle stimulating hormone
GAD glutamic acid decarboxylase
GCS Glasgow Coma Score

GFR glomerular filtration rate
GH growth hormone
GHRH growth hormone releasing hormone
GIK glucose, insulin, and potassium
GIP gastric inhibitory peptide
GLP-1 glucagon-like peptide-1
GMP guanosine monophosphate
GnRH gonadotrophin releasing hormone
(beta)-HCG (beta)-human chorionic gonadotrophin
HDL high-density lipoprotein
HIV human immunodeficiency virus
HLA human leucocyte antigen
HONK hyperosmolar nonketotic diabetic coma
HPA hypothalamo–pituitary–adrenal
HRT hormone replacement therapy
IAA insulin autoantibody
ICA circulating islet cell autoantibody
IDDM insulin-dependent diabetes mellitus
IDL intermediate-density lipoprotein
IFG impaired fasting glucose
IGF-1 insulin-like growth factor-1
IGFBP-3 insulin-like growth factor binding protein-3
IGT impaired glucose tolerance
IPPV intermittent positive-pressure ventilation
IRMA intravascular microvascular abnormality
ITT insulin tolerance test
LDL low-density lipoprotein
LH luteinizing hormone
MAOI monoamine oxidase inhibitor
MEN multiple endocrine neoplasia
MHC major histocompatibility complex
MI myocardial infarction
MIBG meta-iodobenzylguanidine
MODY maturity-onset diabetes of the young
MRI magnetic resonance imaging
MRSA methicillin resistant *Staphylococcus aureus*
NEFA nonesterified fatty acid
NICE National Institute of Clinical Excellence
NIDDM noninsulin-dependent diabetes mellitus
NRT nicotine replacement therapy
NSAID nonsteroidal anti-inflammatory drug
OCP oral contraceptive pill
OGTT oral glucose tolerance test
PAI-1 plasminogen activator inhibitor-1
PCOS polycystic ovarian syndrome
PD-5 phosphodiesterase-5
POF premature ovarian failure
PPARγ peroxisome proliferator activated receptor-gamma
PRA plasma renin activity

PRL prolactin
PSA prostate-specific antigen
PTCA percutaneous angioplasty
PTH parathyroid hormone
PTHrP parathyroid hormone related protein
PVD peripheral vascular disease
RAS renal artery stenosis
RFA radiofrequency ablation
RTH resistance to thyroid hormone
SHBG sex hormone-binding globulin
SIADH syndrome of inappropriate antidiuretic hormone
TBG thyroid binding globulin
TENS transcutaneous electrical nerve stimulation
TFT thyroid function test
TGF-α transforming growth factor-α
TNF-α tumour necrosis factor-α
TRH thyroid releasing hormone
TSH thyroid stimulating hormone
TZD thiazolidinedione
UGDP University Group Diabetes Program
UKPDS United Kingdom Prospective Diabetes Study
VEGF vascular endothelium-derived growth factor
VIP vasointestinal peptide
VLDL very low-density lipoprotein
WHO World Health Organization
ZES Zollinger–Ellison syndrome

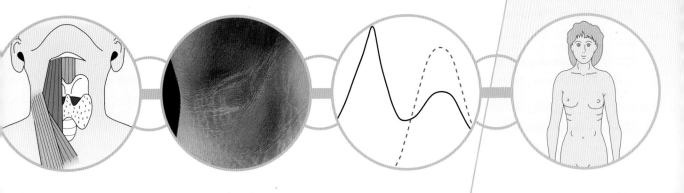

DIABETES

THE IMPACT OF DIABETES

The condition diabetes mellitus may have been in existence for more than three thousand years. The two forms of diabetes were first described in the fifth century AD, one occurring in slim individuals who perished quickly (Type 1 diabetes) and the other in older overweight people who survived for longer (Type 2 diabetes).

By the end of the nineteenth century, Langerhans from Berlin had described small clusters of cells (islets of Langerhans) in the pancreas gland that were later found to be responsible for the production of a glucose-lowering hormone. The greatest break-through in the management of diabetes occurred in 1921 when insulin was discovered at the University of Toronto by the surgeon Frederick Banting and his student Charles Best. This led to insulin being manufactured and used for the treatment of diabetes.

Diabetes mellitus is a condition in which there is a persistent elevation of blood glucose concentration. It can be caused by reduced insulin action and/or insufficient amounts of insulin.

> *The two main types of diabetes are Type 1 diabetes (previously called insulin-dependent diabetes mellitus [IDDM] or juvenile onset diabetes) and Type 2 diabetes (previously called noninsulin dependent diabetes mellitus [NIDDM] or maturity-onset diabetes).*

Type 1 diabetes can occur at any age but more commonly presents in children and young adults. It currently accounts for 5% of diabetes in developing countries and 15% of diabetes in Europe and North America. In most cases it is caused by an autoimmune destruction of the β-cells of the islets of Langerhans cells that are located in the pancreas gland. These cells produce the hormone insulin and their destruction leads to an absence of insulin production and secretion.

Type 2 diabetes has traditionally been considered a disease of the middle-aged or elderly but is now increasingly seen in younger adults and even children, due primarily to increasing rates of obesity. The majority of patients (80–85%) are obese. Obesity and a sedentary lifestyle are thought to be responsible for the dramatic increase in prevalence of this condition. Type 2 diabetes is caused by impaired insulin secretion and by resistance to the action of insulin in peripheral tissues. Features of Types 1 and 2 are presented in *Table 1*.

Diabetes is associated with serious tissue complications resulting from disease of larger (macrovascular) and smaller (microvascular) blood vessels. Microvascular complications occur due to disease of smaller blood vessels, principally affecting the eye (retinopathy), the kidney (nephropathy), and nerves (neuropathy). These strongly relate to the duration of diabetes and the severity of hyperglycaemia.

In the developed world diabetic retinopathy is the most common cause of blindness in those aged <65 years. Diabetic nephropathy is a common cause

---

Table 1 Features of Type 1 and Type 2 diabetes

Type 1 Can occur at almost any age. Rare before 2 years. Most common onset is in childhood and young adult	Type 2 Increasingly common with age. Previously rare before 40 years. Now seen in childhood
❑ Typically slim	❑ Frequently obese (80%) and insulin resistant
❑ Usually symptomatic with weight loss	❑ Symptoms may be mild or absent
❑ Usually no family history	❑ Positive family history commonly found
❑ Hypertension rare at diagnosis	❑ 40% have hypertension at diagnosis
❑ Urinary ketones are usually present at diagnosis	❑ Significant ketosis is rare
❑ Hyperglycaemia responds to insulin only	❑ Hyperglycaemia responds to diet +/- oral agents
❑ Autoantibodies are present at diagnosis	❑ No autoantibodies are found

of renal failure. Peripheral and autonomic neuropathy can both contribute to the development of foot ulceration and increase the risk of amputation. It can also lead to impotence, diarrhoea and vomiting, postural hypotension, and collapse.

Macrovascular complications relate to disease of cardiac, cerebral, and peripheral arteries and is significantly more common in those with diabetes. An increased rate of atherosclerotic disease leads to an excess of ischaemic heart disease, strokes, and lower limb amputation.

The increased morbidity associated with diabetes accounts for more than 5% of total health care costs in Europe. The bulk of this cost relates to the long-term complications rather than the management of the condition itself. It is likely that 90% of the cost relates to disease in patients with Type 2 diabetes.

Life expectancy for a diabetes sufferer is reduced by about 25%. In developed countries, the age-specific mortality rates for those with Type 2 diabetes are approximately twice those of nondiabetic individuals. Most die from cardiovascular disease although nephropathy contributes largely to death rates in Type 1 diabetes.

Type 2 diabetes is increasingly affecting children. In Japan, 80% of childhood diabetes is now due to Type 2 diabetes. In the US this figure is approaching 40%.

INSULIN ACTION

Insulin is synthesized in and secreted from the islets of Langerhans in the endocrine tissue of the pancreas gland. The islets develop from endodermal outgrowths from fetal gut. The normal pancreas has about a million scattered islets of variable size. They comprise only 2% of pancreas volume. The islets contain four main cell types that produce different hormones:
❏ β-cells produce insulin.
❏ α-cells produce glucagons.
❏ δ-cells produce somatostatin.
❏ PP cells produce pancreatic polypeptide.

β-cells are located mainly in the centre of the islet whereas the α- and δ-cells are located towards the periphery. These islet cells interact through direct contact and secretions. The pancreatic islets are innervated with autonomic nerves. Parasympathetic nerves stimulate insulin release while adrenergic sympathetic nerves inhibit insulin and stimulate glucagon. There are additional nerves that stimulate hormone release-producing neuropeptides such as vasointestinal peptide (VIP) and others that inhibit

insulin secretion by producing neuropeptide Y (**1a**).

The main stimulator of insulin production is glucose. The stimulation occurs in a biphasic pattern. There is an acute first phase that lasts several minutes followed by a sustained second phase. The rate of insulin release is controlled by the activity of the enzyme glucokinase. Maximal insulin release occurs at glucose concentrations of 20 mmol/l. Glucose levels below 4 mmol/l, however, do not stimulate insulin release.

Glucose enters the β-cell by the GLUT-2 transporter before being phosphorylated by glucokinase and coupled to insulin release. Glycolysis produces adenosine triphosphate (ATP). This closes ATP sensitive potassium channels, depolarizes the β-cell membrane and leads to an influx of calcium. This leads to granule exocytosis and release of the insulin hormone (**1b**).

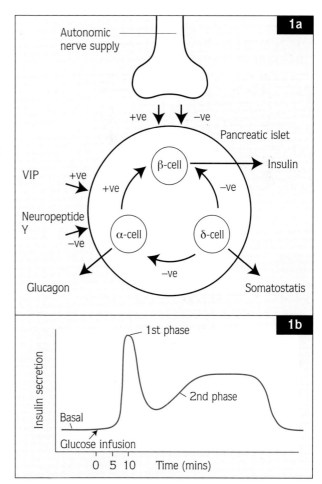

1 Diagram to illustrate pancreatic endocrine function.

Insulin is produced in the β-cells from a single chain precursor called proinsulin. This proinsulin is packaged into vesicles within the Golgi apparatus of the cell and is then mostly converted into insulin and connecting peptide (C-peptide). These two products are released from the cell in secretory granules through microtubules at the cell surface. Insulin consists of two polypeptide chains linked by disulphide bridges. Traditional manufactured insulin products are concentrated and self-associate to form hexamers. These hexamers need to dissociate into six monomers before they can be easily absorbed from subcutaneous tissue (**2**).

Insulin works by binding to cell surface receptors located in the membranes of virtually all mammal cells, α glycoprotein that consists of two extracellular α subunits and two β subunits spanning the cell membrane. When insulin binds to a β subunit this activates the tyrosine kinase enzyme, which in turn activates a complex mechanism of post-receptor signalling that ultimately regulates glucose transport and protein and glycogen synthesis. Glucose is carried into cells by a family of transporter proteins.

Liver cells (hepatocytes), fat cells (adipocytes), and skeletal muscle cells are particularly sensitive to insulin. Brain glucose uptake is not regulated by insulin.

In people without diabetes, blood glucose concentrations are maintained within a narrow range (typically 5–7 mmol/l). This is a balance between glucose release from the liver, glucose uptake into fat cells, skeletal muscle, and peripheral tissues, and absorption from the gastrointestinal tract. Insulin is normally secreted at a low basal level with much higher stimulated levels at meal times. Insulin suppresses glucose output from the liver by inhibiting the breakdown of glycogen (glycogenolysis) and by inhibiting the formation of glucose from other sources such as amino acids, lactate, and glycerol (gluconeogenesis). Only low levels of insulin are required to suppress hepatic glucose output.

Type 1 diabetes leads to a decrease in insulin secretion and an increase in glucagon concentration. The decreased insulin:glucagon ratio increases the production of glucose by the liver and the lack of insulin impairs the utilization of glucose by peripheral tissues, leading to lipolysis in adipose tissue and protein breakdown from muscle. Free fatty acids and amino acids produced from this process are delivered to the liver where there is increased glucose and ketone production through glycogenolysis, gluconeogenesis, and ketosis. Type 1 diabetes also results in an increased secretion of catecholamines such as adrenaline, noradrenaline, growth hormone, cortisol, and vasopressin. These can reduce the sensitivity of peripheral tissues to insulin and increase glucose production from the liver.

THE EPIDEMIOLOGY OF TYPE 1 DIABETES

There is a large geographical variation in the incidence of Type 1 diabetes. In Europe, the frequency increases as from South to North although there is considerable variation between countries. The highest incidence of diabetes is seen in colder autumn and winter months and it is slightly more common in males than females (ratio 1.3:1).

The frequency of Type 1 diabetes is increasing by about 3% per year in most areas of the world.

Environmental factors contribute significantly to the risk of developing Type 1 diabetes but the causative or triggering factor is not known. There is also an inherited risk for developing Type 1 diabetes. One in twenty siblings of affected children will also develop the condition in childhood. It appears that in order to develop Type 1 diabetes an environmental trigger is required to activate an inherited tendency.

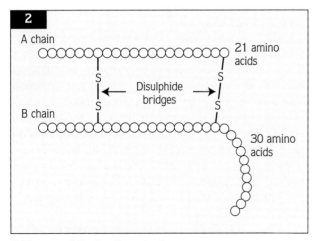

2 Diagram of the insulin molecule.

THE PATHOPHYSIOLOGY OF TYPE 1 DIABETES

The cause of Type 1 diabetes is linked to auto-immunity. The pancreatic islet cells of patients with newly diagnosed Type 1 diabetes contain chronic inflammatory mononuclear cell infiltrate, primarily T lymphocytes and macrophages. As the disease progresses there is complete loss of the β-cells that secrete insulin. This inflammatory reaction can also be identified in the form of circulating autoanti-bodies. In newly diagnosed Type 1 diabetic patients, circulating islet cell autoantibodies (ICAs), glutamic acid decarboxylase (GAD) autoantibodies, insulin autoantibodies (IAAs) and IA-2 antibodies can be found. Islet autoantibodies persist for a period of a few months to a few years before the development of diabetes. However, not all those with antibodies progress to full blown diabetes. Type 1 diabetes is also associated with other organ-specific autoimmune disorders (*Table 2*).

The genetic susceptibility to Type 1 diabetes is most closely linked with human leucocyte antigen (HLA) genes on the short arm of chromosome 6 that lie within the major histocompatibility complex (MHC). More than 95% of UK patients with Type 1 diabetes carry HLA-DR3 and/or DR4 compared with only 50% of nondiabetic individuals. The HLA-DQ6 molecule is associated with a reduced risk of diabetes.

A large number of environmental agents have been implicated in the causation of Type 1 diabetes. Many viruses have been linked. These include mumps, rubella, and Coxsackie B infection. Dietary causes have been implicated in the pathogenesis of diabetes. Of UK Type 1 diabetic patients, 5–10%

have coeliac disease, a gluten-sensitive enteropathy. There may be environmental chemicals that cause Type 1 diabetes. Streptozocin and alloxan can damage the membrane, enzymes, and DNA of the β-cell and can induce a Type 1 diabetes state in rodents. As yet there have been no specific environmental diets or chemicals implicated in humans.

THE EPIDEMIOLOGY OF TYPE 2 DIABETES

The World Health Organization (WHO) has predicted that the global prevalence of Type 2 diabetes will increase from 135 million in 1995 to 300 million in 2025. This increase is affecting both developed and developing countries, with the greatest increases in the poorer, most populous countries. Prevalence rates of 25–50% have been reported in North American Indians, Pacific Islanders, and Australian Aboriginees. In Europe, the prevalence is 3.5% and in the US it is 7%. It affects men and women equally.

THE PATHOPHYSIOLOGY OF TYPE 2 DIABETES AND INSULIN RESISTANCE

The prevalence of Type 2 diabetes increases with age. It is present in 1–2% of those aged 20–40 years but this rises to nearly 20% of those aged over 60 years.

Type 2 diabetes is also linked strongly to obesity. The increased prevalence relates principally to decreased levels of physical activity and increased consumption of calorie-dense food. The risk of developing diabetes increases exponentially with body mass index (BMI). Type 2 diabetes and other cardiovascular risk factors are particularly closely associated with visceral adiposity (abdominal, upper body, and trunk) as opposed to lower body adiposity. There is therefore a strong correlation with an increased waist:hip ratio.

Risk factors for cardiovascular disease are frequently already present when Type 2 diabetes is diagnosed. Hypertension is present in 40% of patients at diagnosis and dyslipidaemia is common. These features are linked by the metabolic defect of insulin resistance. The rate of coronary heart disease, stroke, peripheral vascular disease, and heart failure is increased up to fivefold in patients with Type 2 diabetes. When associated with other biochemical and clinical features, Type 2 diabetes forms part of the syndrome of insulin resistance, also known as the metabolic syndrome.

The metabolic syndrome consists of a combination of cardiovascular risk factors that

---

Table 2 Organ-specific autoimmune disorders associated with diabetes

❑ Primary hypothyroidism
❑ Thyrotoxicosis
❑ Vitiligo
❑ Premature ovarian failure
❑ Pernicious anaemia
❑ Addison's disease

include obesity, dyslipidaemia, insulin rsistance, hypertension, and an increased tendency to thrombosis.

There are also inherited factors linked to the risk of developing Type 2 diabetes. The lifetime risk of developing Type 2 diabetes is 40% if a single parent is similarly affected. Studies of patients with inherited forms of diabetes (maturity-onset diabetes of the young – MODY) have revealed evidence of single gene defects in these individuals. For most cases of Type 2 diabetes, however, there is polygenic inheritance.

Genetic risk may not be the sole reason for familial clustering. The fetal origins hypothesis proposes that Type 2 diabetes results in part from intrauterine malnutrition that increases insulin resistance. Population studies have demonstrated a correlation between low birth weight and the development of Type 2 diabetes and other cardiovascular risk factors. It is likely that genes, ethnicity, and intrauterine factors all contribute to the familial clustering of Type 2 diabetes.

There are defects in both insulin action and secretion in addition to a complex link with the 'insulin resistance syndrome'. The main defects in Type 2 diabetes include a marked delay in both first and second phase insulin responses to meals. There are changes in the normal variability of insulin release and an increase in the circulating proinsulin : insulin ratio.

Resistance to the effects of insulin has been well documented in Type 2 diabetes. However, although insulin resistance is generally high it is also found in some nondiabetic individuals. It cannot, therefore, be entirely responsible for the development of the condition.

OTHER FORMS OF DIABETES

There are a range of conditions and susceptibilities that can lead to other forms of diabetes.

MODY

Maturity-onset diabetes of the young (MODY) is a group of diabetic syndromes that do not usually require insulin therapy. These are caused by a variety of genetic mutations and transmitted in an autosomal dominant fashion. They usually present in childhood and are discussed in the section that relates to childhood diabetes.

LIVER AND PANCREATIC DISEASE

Chronic pancreatitis can lead to an impairment of glucose tolerance or frank diabetes in almost half of sufferers. Histological features include blockage of pancreatic ducts, cysts, fibrosis, and inflammation. Typically one-third of those with diabetes secondary to chronic pancreatitis require insulin therapy. Insulin dose requirements are usually low due to the absence of insulin resistance. Diabetic complications also appear to be less common in this group of patients. **Surgical pancreatectomy** can lead to the development of diabetes if more than 90% of the gland is removed.

Pancreatic carcinoma can present with Type 1 or Type 2 diabetes. Weight loss despite effective treatment, particularly in older patients, should raise suspicion. **Acute pancreatitis**, secondary to gallstone disease or alcohol excess, typically only causes a transient rise in blood glucose.

Haemochromatosis (bronzed diabetes) is an autosomal recessive condition that results in excessive iron absorption and iron deposits in liver, pancreatic islets, skin, and pituitary gland. The clinical features are liver cirrhosis, diabetes, and excessive skin pigmentation. Serum ferritin concentration is raised. A secondary form of this condition is seen in β-thalassaemia due to excessive blood transfusions.

Cystic fibrosis patients are increasingly surviving to adulthood. Diabetes is a common complication of this condition. Insulin is often required although a sulphonylurea drug may suffice in the early stages.

ENDOCRINE DISEASE

Cushing's syndrome leads to insulin resistance due to excessive glucocorticoid production. Cushing's syndrome may be iatrogenic, due to chronic oral or parenteral steroid use. Insulin is required in about 15% of those with steroid-induced diabetes.

Acromegaly leads to insulin resistance through excessive production of growth hormone from a pituitary gland adenoma. Diabetes is seen in 30% of patients with this condition, although many more have a degree of glucose intolerance. **Phaeochromocytoma** results in excessive production of catecholamines, typically adrenaline, noradrenaline, or dopamine. Catecholamines cause insulin resistance, inhibit insulin secretion, stimulate glucagon secretion, stimulate muscle and fat breakdown, and increase glyco-genolysis. **Glucagonoma** is a tumour of the pancreatic islet α-cells that can lead to elevated glucose concentration. It is usually slow growing but ultimately fatal. It can present with thrombosis, psychiatric disturbance, or a classical rash – necrolytic migratory erythema. **Thyrotoxicosis** typically results in delayed post-prandial hyperglycaemia.

Table 3 Secondary causes of diabetes

Pancreatic disease	Chronic pancreatitis, carcinoma of the pancreas, haemachromatosis, cystic fibrosis, pancreatectomy, tropical diabetes
Liver disease	Cirrhosis
Endocrine disease	Cushing's syndrome, acromegaly, phaeochromocytoma, glucagonoma, thyrotoxicosis
Drug-induced disease	Steroid therapy, thiazide diuretics (at higher dose)
Insulin receptor abnormalities	Congenital and acquired lipodystrophies, acanthosis nigricans, leprechaunism
Genetic syndrome	DIDMOAD (Wolfram syndrome), Friedrich's ataxia

INHERITED FORMS OF INSULIN RESISTANCE

Acanthosis nigricans comprises areas of hyper-pigmented, 'velvety' skin and it is typically found in the axillae, back of neck, elbow flexures, and groin. It is associated with insulin resistance (**3**). **Congenital** and **acquired lipodystrophy** is associated with severe insulin resistance. Features can include low body fat, increased muscle bulk, hypertriglyceridaemia, hepatomegaly, and diabetes. **DIDMOAD** (diabetes insipidus, diabetes mellitus, optic atrophy and deafness) is a condition caused by a genetic defect that leads to the conditions outlined in its acronym.

SECONDARY CAUSES OF DIABETES

The secondary causes of diabetes are presented in *Table 3*.

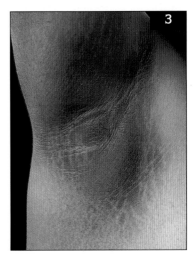

3 Patient with acanthosis nigricans. (Courtesy of Manson Publishing: *Paediatrics and Child Health*, 2007.)

ENDOCRINOLOGY

THE THYROID GLAND – STRUCTURE AND FUNCTION

The thyroid gland develops from the endoderm of the floor of the pharynx and the lateral pharyngeal pouches. It gives rise to the thyroglossal duct that runs from the base of the tongue to the thyroid isthmus. The gland lies anteriorly, within the pre-tracheal fascia of the neck. Posteriorly it is anchored to the trachea so that the gland rises during swallowing. Anteriorly are the strap muscles of the neck. The gland has a midline isthmus that sits below the cricoid cartilage and two larger lateral lobes that overlie the thyroid cartilage (**4**).

The gland consists of a large number of follices surrounded by capillary networks and divided by fibrous septa. Within the follicles is colloid material containing thyroglobulin. The thyroid hormones thyroxine (T_4) and tri-iodothyronine (T_3) are synthesized from follicular cells (thyrocytes) from

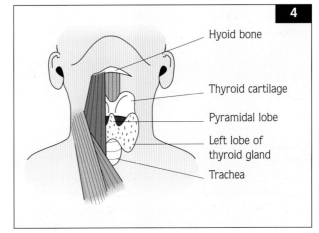

Hyoid bone
Thyroid cartilage
Pyramidal lobe
Left lobe of thyroid gland
Trachea

4 Diagram of the thyroid gland.

thyroglobulin and secreted under the control of thyroid stimulating hormone (TSH) produced from the anterior pituitary gland. Thyroid hormone production begins as early as 10 weeks fetal gestation. Thyroid hormone concentration is tightly controlled by feedback mechanisms of the hypothalamo–pituitary–thyroid axis.

Thyroid hormones contain large amounts of iodine. Inorganic iodide enters the thyroid gland and is oxidized by a peroxidase enzyme at the cell–colloid interface before forming iodothyronine. The thyroid secretes all available T_4 but only 20% of T_3. The remainder is formed peripherally from the deiodination of T_4. Some T_4 is converted to metabolically inactive reverse T_3 (rT_3).

T_4 and T_3 in the blood are mostly bound to plasma proteins. T_4 is predominantly bound to thyroid binding globulin (TBG) and other plasma proteins, including albumin. Thyroid status correlates more closely, however, with free, rather than bound, thyroid hormone levels since it is the free hormone that is metabolically active. Most laboratories now measure free thyroid hormones since a number of states can increase levels of TBG, leading to spuriously high levels of measured bound thyroid hormone (*Table 4*).

Thyroid hormone levels are controlled by feedback mechanisms (5). Thyroid releasing hormone (TRH) stimulates the synthesis and secretion of TSH. TSH from the pituitary stimulates the thyroid to secrete the thyroid hormones T_4 and, to a lesser extent, T_3. T_4 and T_3 act directly to reduce the synthesis and secretion of TSH.

Situated within the thyroid gland are also parafollicular cells (c-cells) that secrete calcitonin, a hormone that plays a role in bone metabolism.

THE PARATHYROID GLANDS – STRUCTURE AND FUNCTION

The parathyroid glands are oval structures that weigh about 30 mg each. There are usually four of them and they lie on the posterior surface of the thyroid gland. Normally they are symmetrically arranged, with the two superior parathyroids lying about 1 cm above the point where the inferior thyroid artery enters the thyroid gland. The two inferior (lower) parathyroid glands lie 1 cm below this point. There is variation in the number and location of glands. More than four glands are present in 5% of people. Parathyroid glands can be found high at the level of the thyroid cartilage or hyoid bone. They have also been found low at a level of the inferior pole of the thyroid or manubrium and in the chest. They can be either within or outside the fibrous capsule of the thyroid. Extracapsular parathyroids are not constrained and

---

Table 4 Conditions that lead to raised thyroid binding globulin

❏ Pregnancy; genetically determined
❏ Exogenous oestrogen, e.g. oral contraceptive pill
❏ Chronic liver disease
❏ Acute intermittent porphyria
❏ Hepatitis A

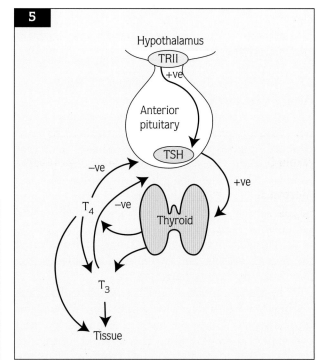

5 Diagram of the control and secretion of thyroid hormones.

may expand downwards into the mediastinum. The superior parathyroids are derived from the fourth branchial pouches and the inferior parathyroids from the third branchial pouches.

Branches of the inferior thyroid artery supply the parathyroid glands. The glands drain into the plexus of veins on the anterior surface of the thyroid comprising the superior, middle, and inferior thyroid veins. Histologically the glands contain a number of cells, most importantly the chief cells that secrete parathyroid hormone (PTH). PTH is an 84-aminoacid polypeptide that is secreted from the parathyroid gland in response to hypocalcaemia. It has a number of effects:

❑ Bone resorption by increasing osteoclastic activity, therefore mobilizing calcium from bone.
❑ Reabsorption of calcium at the distal convoluted tubule in the kidney.
❑ Increased synthesis of 1-25 dihydroxy-cholecalciferol (the active form of Vitamin D) in the kidney, leading to calcium reabsorption from the gastrointestinal system.

As calcium levels rise there is a negative feedback loop that inhibits further PTH release, thus maintaining a balanced calcium level.

Calcium is an integral part of many biological systems. It is involved in muscle contraction–relaxation, clotting, mitotic division, and synaptic transmission. Calcium in the body is found in three forms with most present in the bony skeleton:

❑ Calcium combined with phosphorus in the skeleton (98%).
❑ Calcium bound to proteins such as albumin (1%).
❑ Ionized calcium, which is physiologically active (1%).

The physiologically important ionized calcium has to be closely regulated (normal range 2.2–2.6 mmol/l) and homeostasis of normal calcium levels is controlled by osteoclastic activity, gastrointestinal absorption of calcium, renal excretion of calcium, and the effects of PTH. The effects of hormones on calcium regulation are shown in *Table 5*.

THE ADRENAL GLANDS – STRUCTURE AND FUNCTION

An adrenal gland sits above both left and right kidney. Each weighs 4–5 g and consists of a central medulla surrounded by a thick cortex that comprises 90% of the gland volume. Blood supply is primarily from aorta and renal arteries. Venous drainage is into the inferior vena cava on the right and the left renal vein on the left.

The adrenal medulla produces the catecholamines adrenaline, noradrenaline, and dopamine.

The adrenal cortex is composed of three zones, an outer zona glomerulosa, a zona fasciculata, and an inner zona reticularis. The zona fasciculata and zona

Table 5 Effects of hormones on calcium regulation

Hormone	Bone	Kidney	Gut
Parathyroid hormone	Increases release of calcium and phosphate	Increases reabsorption of calcium. Reduces reabsorption of phosphate	
Vitamin D		Decreases reabsorption of calcium	Increases uptake of calcium and phosphate
Calcitonin	Reduces release of calcium and phosphate	Decreases reabsorption of calcium and phosphate	

reticularis synthesize the glucocorticoid cortisol and androgens (principally androstenedione, dihydro-epiandrostenedione [DHEA] and DHEA sulphate) and are closely regulated by adrenocorticotrophic hormone (ACTH) from the anterior pituitary gland. The zona glomerulosa synthesizes aldosterone. These hormones are synthesized from cholesterol via a number of enzyme-controlled steps (6).

Cortisol secretion is episodic but has a circadian rhythm, peaking in the sixth to eighth hours of sleep and declining at wakening (7). It increases during times of physical stress. Cortisol exhibits a negative feedback on the secretion of both corticotrophin releasing hormone (CRH) from the hypothalamus and ACTH from the pituitary. Cortisol has a metabolic effect on most tissues. It is catabolic and increases hepatic gluconeogenesis and lipolysis and inhibits glucose uptake in muscle and fat. It has profound effects on protein catabolism and the immune system. Excessive cortisol, however, has a deleterious effect on bone, skin, growth, and most organ systems.

Adrenal androgens are precursors for peripheral conversion to testosterone and dihydrotestosterone. Their contribution to the androgen pool is much greater in women than in men.

The mineralocorticoid aldosterone is predominantly produced as part of the renin–angiotensin axis (8) although it is regulated in part by ACTH (<10%). It is produced in the zona glomerulosa and is responsible for electrolyte regulation and control of extracellular volume. Renin is secreted by arteriolar smooth muscle cells in the juxtaglomerular apparatus within the renal cortex. Renin converts angiotensinogen in blood to angiotensin I. Renin release is controlled by pressure change in the afferent arteriole, sympathetic tone, solute concentrations, and local prostaglandin release. Angiotensin II is generated from angiotensin I by angiotensin-converting enzyme (ACE). Angiotensin II is a vasoconstrictor that also directly stimulates aldosterone release from the adrenal cortex.

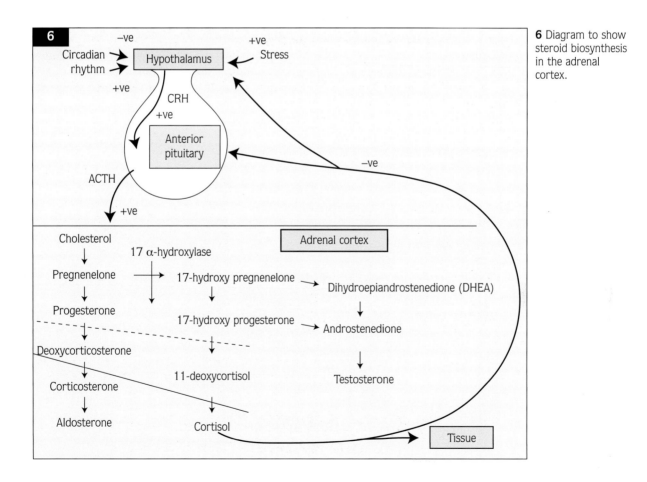

6 Diagram to show steroid biosynthesis in the adrenal cortex.

The adrenal medulla arises from the sympathetic nervous system and holds a large number of chromaffin cells with granules that contain the catecholamines dopamine, adrenaline, and nor-adrenaline. These catabolic hormones are secreted in reponse to exercise, physical stress, hypoglycaemia, and anoxia. Release is mediated by acetylcholine from the terminals of preganglionic sympathetic nerve fibres. These hormones act directly on blood vessels, heart, kidney, gut, liver, adipose tissue, skin, and bronchioles.

THE PITUITARY GLAND – STRUCTURE AND FUNCTION

The pituitary gland is situated in the pituitary fossa. It is continuous with the pituitary stalk of the hypothalamus above. It is surrounded by the sphenoid sinus below and by cavernous sinuses on either side. Embryologically and functionally the pituitary gland can be divided into two sections, the anterior and posterior pituitary (9).

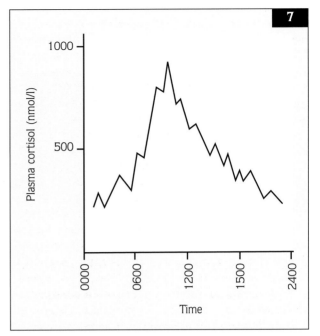

7 Graph to show the circadian nature of cortisol secretion.

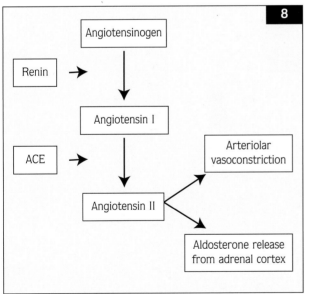

8 Diagram to illustrate the renin–angiotensin axis controlling mineralocorticoid production.

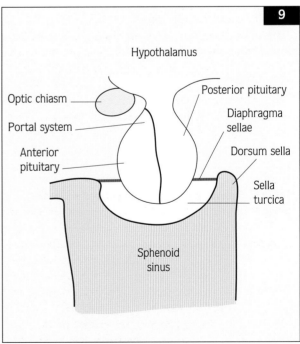

9 Diagram to show the anatomic relationships of the pituitary gland.

The anterior pituitary gland is supplied by hypothalamohypophyseal portal veins. It develops from the pouch of Rathke below.

> *The anterior pituitary gland is responsible for the secretion of six major hormones:*
> ❏ *Growth hormone (GH).*
> ❏ *Luteinizing hormone (LH).*
> ❏ *Follicle stimulating hormone (FSH).*
> ❏ *Thyroid stimulating hormone (TSH).*
> ❏ *Adrenocorticotrophic hormone (ACTH).*
> ❏ *Prolactin (PRL).*

The secretion of these hormones is controlled by stimulating and inhibitory factors produced in the hypothalamus and secreted into portohypophyseal blood vessels (*Table 6*).

The posterior pituitary gland derives from the forebrain. It is responsible for the secretion of antidiuretic hormone (ADH; vasopressin) and oxytocin. These hormones are synthesized in the supraoptic and paraventricular nuclei of the hypothalamus and are transported as neurosecretory granules via neurohypophyseal tracts to the posterior pituitary gland where they are released into the circulation. These hormones are not bound to plasma proteins and have a short half-life.

In women, oxytocin results in contraction of the pregnant uterus and breast duct smooth muscle. It leads to breast milk ejection during breast-feeding. ADH is a nonapeptide that is primarily released in response to changes in osmolality detected by hypothalamic osmoreceptors. This hormone acts on the renal collecting duct and ascending loop of Henle. It increases water permeability so that water diffuses to the interstitial medulla by osmosis. It therefore enables the kidneys to concentrate urine.

LIPID METABOLISM

Cholesterol and triglycerides are insoluble and transported between the gut, liver, and peripheral tissues as soluble lipoproteins. They include high-density (HDL), low-density (LDL), intermediate-density (IDL) and very low density (VLDL) lipoproteins.

Chylomicrons are large particles consisting mainly of triglycerides and are synthesized in the mucosa of the small intestine. LDLs are the major cholesterol-carrying lipoprotein. The pathways of lipid metabolism are shown in figure 10.

Table 6 Hypothalamic releasing hormones and pituitary hormones

Hypothalamic hormone	Effect on anterior pituitary
TRH	Increases TSH and prolactin secretion
GnRH	Increases LH and FSH secretion
GHRH	Increases GH secretion
CRH	Increases ACTH secretion
Dopamine inhibitory peptide	Reduces prolactin secretion
Somatostatin	Inhibits GH and TSH secretion

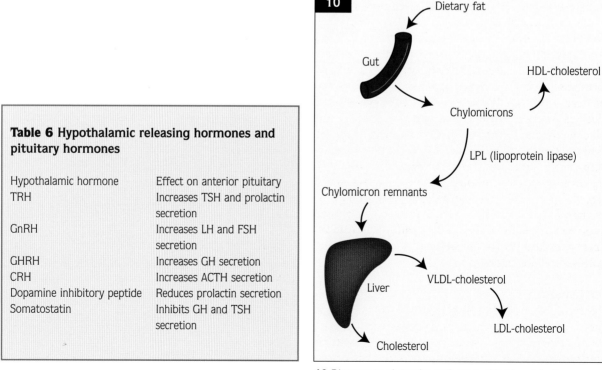

10 Diagram to show the pathways of lipid metabolism.

THE REPRODUCTIVE ORGANS – STRUCTURE AND FUNCTION

THE FEMALE

The ovaries are paired structures weighing 4–8 g that are situated behind the peritoneum, attached to the posterior surface of the broad ligament by a fold of peritoneum. They are attached to the uterus by the broad ligament and lie in close association with the fallopian tubes.

Oestradiol is the most potent oestrogen and is produced by ovarian granulosa cells. The ovaries also produce androgens, some of which are converted to oestradiol by the aromatase enzyme. In ovulating women, the corpus luteum produces progesterone in the second half (luteal phase) of the menstrual cycle. Oestradiol has widespread effects. It is essential for follicular and oocyte maturation, growth of the uterus and vagina, stimulation of cervical mucous, and development of the endometrium. It also contributes to libido, breast growth, musculoskeletal growth, and the female pattern of fat distribution. It stimulates the production of sex hormone-binding globulin (SHBG) from the liver to which it is mostly bound in the serum.

Progesterone helps to maintain pregnancy by inhibiting uterine activity and helps amplify the LH surge at ovulation. In the first half (follicular phase) of the menstrual cycle, oestradiol levels peak a day or two before ovulation. Progesterone levels rise with the LH surge shortly before ovulation.

FSH and LH stored in the anterior pituitary are stimulated by pulsatile gonadotropin releasing hormone (GnRH) secretion from the hypothalamus but are controlled primarily by oestrogen and progesterone secretion. Towards the end of the follicular phase FSH levels rise as negative feedback from ovarian hormones falls. As oestradiol secretion increases during the follicular phase there is a sudden LH surge triggered 36 hours before ovulation which lasts 48 hours. This stimulates final maturation of the graafian follicle to release its oocyte. There is a small accompanying FSH surge. The gonadotrophin levels quickly reduce to low levels in the presence of oestradiol and progesterone (**11**).

THE MALE

The two testes each average 2.5–4.5 cm in length. They are located within the scrotum which serves as a protective envelope and helps maintain a testicular temperature that is 2°C below abdominal temperature. The testes contain two major components, the Leydig cells and the seminiferous tubules. The masculinizing hormone testosterone and other androgens are produced in the interstitial Leydig cells that lie alongside the seminiferous tubules. The seminiferous tubules make up most of the testicular volume and comprise the germ cells and Sertoli cells. A number of local hormones produced here support spermatogenesis and prevent female sex organ development. Spermatogenesis occurs here. The process of spermatogenesis takes 2–3 months.

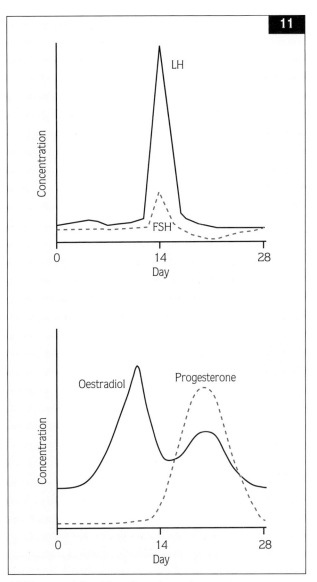

11 The gonadotrophin and ovarian cycles.

The regulation of testosterone production is through the pulsatile secretion of the hypothalamic hormone GnRH which stimulates gonadotrophin production (LH and FSH) from the anterior pituitary gland. The rate of frequency of these pulses determines whether more LH or FSH is produced.

❑ *LH binds to Leydig cell receptors to stimulate the secretion and synthesis of testosterone.*
❑ *FSH binds to Sertoli cell receptors to stimulate the production of fluid, inhibin, and hormones required for spermatogenesis.*

Pituitary gonadotrophin secretion is regulated by testosterone and inhibin produced in the testes through a complex system of negative feedback. Testosterone is mostly bound to albumin and SHBG. The free portion (3%) is metabolically active. It is converted in peripheral tissues to the more potent dihydrotestosterone and is essential for male virilization and sexual development.

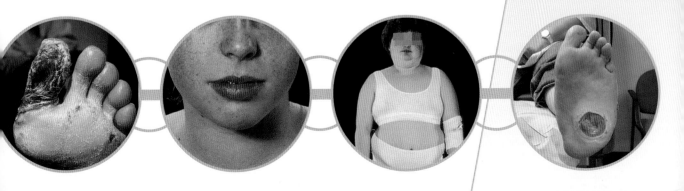

DIABETES

DIAGNOSIS

The characteristic and diagnostic feature of diabetes is a chronic elevation of plasma glucose concentration.

UK diagnostic criteria for diabetes:
❏ Fasting plasma glucose (FPG): 7.0 mmol/l or greater.
❏ Random plasma glucose: 11.1 mmol/l or greater.
❏ Following an oral glucose tolerance test (OGTT), 2 hours post 75 g glucose load: 11.1 mmol/l or greater.

The diagnosis can be made from a single plasma glucose level in a patient with symptoms. Typical symptoms of diabetes are thirst, polyuria, lethargy, weight loss, and blurred vision.

In an asymptomatic patient two abnormal results are required from two separate days. An elevated HbA1c, glycosuria, or elevated capillary finger-prick glucose does not satisfy the diagnostic criteria for diabetes. To obtain a fasting plasma glucose, the patient should be starved for 8 hours and the test carried out in the morning. The patient should only drink water during this period and should usually avoid medical treatment until after the test has been performed.

The OGTT requires 75 g glucose to be dissolved in 250 ml of water and then ingested. The patient should be fasting. Venous blood is sampled before and 120 minutes after ingestion. An OGTT should be considered in those with impaired fasting or random glucose.

Impaired fasting glucose (IFG) and impaired glucose tolerance (IGT) are intermediate categories of hyperglycaemia.
❏ IFG is defined as a fasting plasma glucose >6 mmol/l but less than 7 mmol/l.
❏ IGT is a plasma glucose ≥7.8 mmol/l but <11.1 mmol/l at 2 hours post OGTT.

False positive diagnoses of diabetes or IFG may occur if the subject has been inadequately prepared for a fasting test. Using the fasting concentration alone may miss some individuals with diabetes since the initial phase of diabetes involves impairment of the first phase postprandial insulin release. Individuals with IGT may have fasting glucose concentrations that lie within the normal, IFG, or diabetic range.

Using the fasting glucose method is imperfect but it simplifies the diagnostic process and is adequate in most clinical settings.

PRESENTATION

Typically Type 1 diabetes presents either subacutely with a classic triad of symptoms, or more acutely with illness and ketoacidosis when the initial symptoms have not been recognized. Although there may have been a significant deterioration in β-cell function for up to 3 years, the presentation is usually fairly acute, with preceding symptoms lasting for a period of up to several weeks. The triad of symptoms includes:
❏ Polyuria: due to the effect of osmotic diuresis that occurs when blood glucose levels exceed the renal threshold.
❏ Thirst and polydipsia: due to the resulting loss of fluid and electrolytes.
❏ Weight loss: due to fluid depletion and the accelerated loss of fat and muscle that results from insulin deficiency.

Type 2 diabetes can present in many different ways, from the asymptomatic chance discovery to the life-threatening hyperosmolar nonketotic diabetic coma (HONK). Most patients will have had the condition for some time prior to diagnosis. Typical symptoms include thirst, polyuria, fatigue, and blurred vision. Weight loss is more typical of Type 1 diabetes. Symptoms are frequently absent. An individual may present with microvascular or macrovascular complications as presented in *Table 7*. Alternatively, the patient may present with an infection; common presenting conditions include genital candidiasis (thrush), cellulitis, or a urinary tract infection. Additional eye disorders (cataract and glaucoma) may also lead to the diagnosis of diabetes being made.

ACUTE/EMERGENCY DIABETES CARE

In additon to its chronic complications, diabetes can present acutely with problems that relate directly to blood glucose levels:
❏ Hypoglycaemia.
❏ Diabetic ketoacidosis (DKA).
❏ Hyperosmolar nonketotic states (e.g. HONK).
❏ Lactic acidosis.

HYPOGLYCAEMIA

Hypoglycaemia is a common side-effect of treatment for diabetes. It causes a great deal of anxiety for patients because it is unpleasant and dangerous.

❏ Biochemical hypoglycaemia is defined as a plasma glucose <2.8 mmol/l.

❏ Clinical hypoglycaemia can occur at a lower or higher glucose concentration. It may be mild (self-managed) or severe (requiring either the assistance of a third person or hospital admission).

In Type 1 diabetes mild hypoglycaemia occurs on average twice weekly and is more common on weekdays than weekends. Severe hypoglycaemia occurs in 10% of Type 1 diabetic patients per year. The tighter the glucose control the more likely that hypoglycaemia will occur. The hypoglycaemic risk is lower for those with Type 2 diabetes, even when insulin-treated; the incidence of severe hypoglycaemia is 2.3% per year. In tablet-controlled patients this figure falls to 0.025% per year. However, one in six tablet-controlled patients will still experience mild hypoglycaemia during the first year of therapy.

Pathophysiology of hypoglycaemia

In those without diabetes, fasting blood glucose does not typically fall into the hypoglycaemic range. It is prevented from doing so by a fall in the insulin:glucagon ratio in portal circulation. This results in an increase of hepatic glucose output through increased glycogen breakdown and gluco-neogenesis.

Individuals who are treated with insulin or β-cell stimulating drugs such as the sulphonylureas cannot switch off insulin production despite falling glucose concentration. There continues to be suppression of glucose output despite peripheral uptake of glucose. The brain does not have its own supply of glucose and is critically dependent upon circulating glucose. In response to impending hypoglycaemia, it activates counter-regulatory hormone responses.

There is an increase in glucagon production from pancreatic α-cells. This increases hepatic glucose output through glycogenolysis and then gluconeo-genesis. Adrenaline is released from the sympathetic nervous system and this inhibits hepatic glucose output and reduces peripheral glucose uptake. Other stress hormones (cortisol and growth hormone [GH]) are produced more slowly and become important where there is prolonged hypoglycaemia.

Table 7 Micro- and macrovascular complications of diabetes

Microvascular complication	Presentation
Retinopathy	Visual impairment or a chance discovery
Nephropathy	Proteinuria, hypertension or nephrotic syndrome
Neuropathy	Painful sensory peripheral neuropathy, mononeuropathy, carpal tunnel syndrome, amyotrophy, or foot ulceration

Macrovascular complication	Presentation
Coronary	Angina or myocardial infarction
Cerebral	Stroke, transient ischaemic attacks
Peripheral	Intermittent claudication, rest pain, ischaemic leg

Symptoms and signs of hypoglycaemia

The symptoms and signs of hypoglycaemia can be broadly divided into two main types: autonomic and neuroglycopenic (*Table 8*).

Seizures accompany 10% of severe hypoglycaemic episodes and these are more common in children. They tend to be generalized grand mal events. Hypoglycaemia is a likely cause of seizures if occurring overnight in children with good glucose control.

Focal neurological signs can be seen in severe hypoglycaemia and this can give the appearance of a hemiplegic stroke. However, symptoms and signs resolve quickly on correcting the hypoglycaemia. In severe cases cerebral oedema leads to death or a persistent vegetative state secondary to cerebral atrophy. There is evidence in the very young (<5 years) that episodes of hypoglycaemia may lead to chronic cognitive and intellectual impairment.

The causes of hypoglycaemia

> *The risk of severe hypoglycaemia is increased with tight blood glucose control and in Type 1 patients who have had a long duration of diabetes.*

A single severe hypoglycaemic episode will impair further counter-regulatory responses to hypoglycaemia for more than a week. Frequent mild episodes of hypoglycaemia also impair this response and result in a loss of autonomic warning symptoms. To correct this loss an intensive training programme to avoid hypoglycaemia is often helpful. This involves intensive education and frequent blood glucose testing. Subjects are taught the importance of frequent snacking and the effects of lifestyle and insulin dose adjustment on blood glucose concentration.

The newer insulin analogues may be useful tools in reducing the frequency of hypoglycaemia.

Autonomic warning symptoms are reduced in those with a long duration of diabetes (>15 years). The glucagon response is lost first, leaving patients to rely upon neuroglycopenic symptoms. At a later stage the adrenergic response is also reduced. This delays the return to normoglycaemia after hypoglycaemia.

With insulin-treated diabetes the major causes of acute hypoglycaemia are too much insulin, inadequate food intake, excessive exercise, or alcohol ingestion (*Table 9*). Too much insulin may be secondary to a poor understanding of the appropriateness of an insulin dose or a miscalculation of its effect, although there is an inherent variability in glucose concentration that makes the precise calculation of an insulin dose difficult. Insulin absorption may be increased if insulin is administered intramuscularly, the ambient temperature is high, or the injection site is more central (abdomen > arm > thigh). If insulin is injected into sites of lipo-

---

Table 8 Symptoms and signs of hypoglycaemia

Classification	Pathogenesis	Symptoms
Autonomic	Occur as a result of activating the sympathetic nervous system with adrenaline release from the adrenal medulla. These symptoms are usually triggered at a plasma glucose concentration <3 mmol/l	Early autonomic symptoms include hunger, sweating, tremor, anxiety, and palpitations. These should warn sufferers of approaching hypoglycaemia and stimulate the intake of food.
Neuroglycopenic	These may precede autonomic symptoms in some, and this can make it difficult for symptoms to be recognized and interpreted	Light-headedness, confusion, headache, irritability or tiredness are early symptoms. This can lead to aggression, slurred speech, and lack of coordination. Severe hypoglycaemia leads to drowsiness, seizures, and coma.

hypertrophy insulin absorption will be more erratic. With many diabetes regimes it is important to ensure regular energy intake during the day, particularly when insulin is injected twice daily. Delayed or missed meals are a common cause of hypoglycaemia.

Alcohol is implicated in 20% of hospital admissions with hypoglycaemia. Even in small amounts it causes a delayed hypoglycaemic effect, probably through its effects on counter-regulatory hormone production. This is most commonly seen in the early hours of the morning. It is important for those who have consumed alcohol during the evening to ensure that someone checks to see how they are early the following morning. Alcohol may impair awareness and cognitive function so that appropriate action is not taken to correct hypoglycaemia.

Newly diagnosed Type 1 patients have an increased risk of hypoglycaemia due to the fall in insulin requirements that occurs during the initial months (honeymoon period). Those with pancreatic disease may have an increased risk of severe and prolonged hypoglycaemia, particularly if they are dependent upon alcohol. Those with renal failure are at increased risk of hypoglycaemia since insulin is partly catabolized by the kidneys. Clinicians should be alert to this possibility when glucose control is improving without explanation. Secondary Addison's disease, hypopituitarism, and hypothyroidism are other medical causes.

Rarely, hypoglycaemia is secondary to deliberate insulin or sulphonylurea overdose. Typically, insulin overdose occurs in patients with underlying psychiatric illness. Occasionally it is taken by friends or relatives of diabetic patients and rarely has been deliberately administered to others. Nonselective beta-blockers may delay the recovery from hypoglycaemia but rarely lead to clinical problems.

There is increasing evidence that overnight hypoglycaemia in Type 1 diabetes is more common than previously thought. This may be particularly problematic in children. The newer short-acting insulin analogues are less likely to lead to overnight and daytime hypoglycaemia than traditional short-acting insulin preparations. There is also evidence that use of the longer-acting insulin analogue glargine may be less likely to cause overnight hypoglycaemia than traditional intermediate-acting insulin preparations. A continuous insulin infusion pump may help in some patients with recurrent hypoglycaemia. Missed or delayed meals are a common cause for hypoglycaemia in tablet-controlled patients (*Table 9*).

Sulphonylurea-induced hypoglycaemia, particularly when glucose control is tight, is a common complication. It is is more common in the elderly and in those with renal or hepatic failure. Long-acting sulphonylurea drugs such as glibenclamide should be avoided in the elderly since they increase the risk and duration of hypoglycaemia.

Nondiabetic hypoglycaemia

Spontaneous hypoglycaemia is classified as either fasting hypoglycaemia, occurring many hours after the ingestion of food, typically at night or early morning, or reactive hypoglycaemia, occurring within 5 hours of food ingestion. It is important to determine the timing of hypoglycaemic symptoms since reactive hypoglycaemia does not necessarily signify underlying disease. Reactive hypoglycaemia may be idiopathic or may precede the development of diabetes mellitus. It is also seen following gastrectomy (late dumping) occurring 1–3 hours after food consumption. Causes of nondiabetic hypoglycaemia include:
- Acute liver or renal failure.
- Septicaemia.
- Starvation.
- Insulinoma.
- Fibrosarcoma.
- Mesothelioma.
- Hepatocellular carcinoma.

Table 9 **Causes of hypoglycaemia in diabetic patients**

- Excessive insulin administration
- Tight blood glucose control
- Missed or delayed meals
- Exercise
- Alcohol
- Changes in injection sites
- Sulphonylurea drugs
- Coexistent endocrine disease (Addison's disease, hypothyroidism, hypopituitarism)

❑ Hormone deficiency (cortisol, growth hormone [GH] or adrenocorticotrophic hormone [ACTH] deficiency).

❑ Autoimmune (insulin antibodies – rare).

❑ Drug-induced overdose of insulin, sulphonylureas, alcohol, quinine, or aspirin.

❑ Inborn errors of metabolism.

Investigation of nondiabetic hypoglycaemia

If deliberate overdose or malicious administration of insulin or a sulphonylurea is suspected, blood should be taken from the intravenous cannula prior to glucose infusion. This blood should be kept for analysis of plasma glucose, insulin and C-peptide concentration. Urine should be assayed for the presence of sulphonylurea drugs. Screening investigations should include chest X-ray, liver function tests, serum cortisol (followed by synacthen test if indicated), and fasting glucose, insulin, and C-peptide. An overnight (>15 hour) fast can be used to help screen for the presence of an insulinoma (see later).

DIABETIC KETOACIDOSIS (DKA)

Diabetic ketoacidosis (DKA) is a state of severe uncontrolled diabetes with hyperglycaemia, ketonaemia, and metabolic acidosis.

DKA has an annual incidence of about 1 in 200 people with diabetes. It is more common in females (2:1) and occurs most commonly in children and least commonly in older adults (age >30 years). It is a recurring problem for 1 in 7 patients. Before the development of insulin, DKA was fatal but it now leads to death in less than 10% of cases. There is a greater risk for older people (>50 years) where the fatality rates approach 20%. This increased risk is predominantly due to comorbid illnesses.

DKA occurs as a result of insulin deficiency. Insulin deficiency leads to increased glycogenolysis and gluconeogenesis and reduced peripheral uptake of glucose. The increase in plasma glucose causes an osmotic diuresis, with increased urine output and thirst. In states of insulin deficiency, glucagon is raised. This further increases hepatic gluconeogenesis and hyperglycaemia. It also leads to lipolysis resulting in the liberation of free fatty acids that are converted to ketone bodies in the liver. These lead to vomiting and a metabolic acidosis. Together with the osmotic diuresis this results in dehydration and electrolyte imbalances.

A typical DKA may result in a loss of 6 litres of water, 1000 mmol/l of sodium, and 500 mmol/l of potassium plus calcium, chloride, phosphate and other mineral losses.

Common precipitants for DKA are infection, inadequate or missed insulin doses, and new diagnosis. DKA may be seen in conjunction with major medical conditions such as myocardial infarction and stroke. Concomitant medical conditions are more common in the elderly (around 50%). In younger patients, deliberate omission of insulin may form part of a stress-related condition or an eating disorder.

Clinical features

DKA develops over a period of 12–24 hours. If suspected, a rapid history, physical examination, and bedside tests should be performed after emergency management.

Symptoms include thirst, polyuria, visual blurring, breathlessness, nausea/vomiting, abdominal pain, and drowsiness. There may additional symptoms secondary to an infection or other medical condition.

❑ Thirst, polyuria, and visual blurring are due to the effects of hyperglycaemia.

❑ Breathlessness is due to deep, rapid 'kussmaul' breathing– a respiratory response to the metabolic acidosis.

❑ Abdominal pain is epigastric or generalized and responds to treatment of DKA. Drowsiness correlates with raised plasma osmolarity.

❑ Physical examination may reveal dehydration, hypotension, tachycardia, acetone breath, reduced conscious level, and 'kussmaul' breathing.

❑ Abdominal examination may reveal a rigid abdomen and absent bowel sounds. Acetone can be detected on the breath as it carries an odour of 'pear drops'.

Immediate investigations should include the following:

❑ Plasma glucose. A bedside sample can be measure using a meter but this should be confirmed with a laboratory sample.

❑ Plasma urea and electrolytes. Urea will be raised due to dehydration. With insulin deficiency and acidosis, potassium leaks from intracellular sites and the plasma potassium concentration may be raised despite urinary and gastric loss. Plasma sodium may be low. Urinary losses contribute to this. Also, hyperglycaemia leads to excessively dilute plasma since there is osmotic movement of water from intra- to extracellular space.

❑ Urinary ketones. This is best measured with 'Ketostix' or an alternative nitroprusside based reagent.

❑ Arterial blood gases or venous bicarbonate. This helps assess the severity of acidosis.
❑ Septic screen. Urine and blood cultures to exclude underlying infection.
❑ Echocardiogram +/– cardiac enzymes. These will exclude myocardial infarction and may not be necessary in younger patients.
❑ Chest X-ray. Carried out if lung infection is a possibility.

Other investigations may be performed that can be misleading in DKA. A white cell count may be elevated to 20 000 × 10^9/l and the serum amylase may be elevated threefold. Serum triglycerides may also be significantly raised, giving the blood sample a milky appearance.

HYPEROSMOLAR NONKETOTIC DIABETIC COMA (HONK)

Hyperosmolar nonketotic diabetic coma (HONK) is a hyperglycaemic emergency that is typically seen in patients with Type 2 diabetes. It generally occurs in older patients (aged >50 years) and is slightly more common in women than in men. It is less common than DKA but can be the presenting feature of Type 2 diabetes in 30% of cases.

HONK is similar to DKA in that it presents with hyperglycaemia, dehydration, and electrolyte disturbances. The management is similar. Unlike DKA, patients with HONK do not suffer with ketoacidosis. This is probably due to the effect of higher insulin and lower counter-regulatory hormone concentrations, preventing hepatic production of ketones.

> *HONK usually presents with a gradual onset of symptoms over a period of several days.*

Typically the picture is of an elderly patient who has become increasingly drowsy. Kussmaul breathing is not present and vomiting is less common than with DKA. It is characterized by marked hyperglycaemia and dehydration. This is due to a more prolonged period of worsening control associated with persistent osmotic diuresis. Frequently, thirst sensation is not fully intact in the elderly who may find it less easy to access adequate fluid. Plasma glucose and osmolarity are significantly raised and plasma sodium may also be elevated. The conscious level of the patient relates closely to the plasma osmolarity and the severity of dehydration.

> *Precipitating factors may be co-morbid ill health, (often sepsis or vascular disease), a recent surgical procedure, or drug-induced (steroid or thiazide treatment).*

Other physical findings include seizures and focal neurological abnormalities. These should resolve upon treatment. In addition to markedly raised plasma glucose (>40 mmol/l), raised plasma osmolarity (>300 mOsmol/l), and raised sodium (variable) there may be other biochemical findings. Serum potassium may be elevated initially but falls with the initiation of treatment to hypokalaemic levels. Urea concentration is elevated due to dehydration. Bicarbonate may be low if there is lactic acidosis.

LACTIC ACIDOSIS

This rare complication may be seen in diabetic patients with ischaemic heart disease. It can also be seen as part of DKA or in Type 2 patients taking metformin therapy. Metformin-induced lactic acidosis is usually associated with renal or hepatic failure.

Lactic acidosis should be suspected in severely ill diabetic patients with a metabolic acidosis that cannot be entirely attributed to ketosis. Calculation of the anion gap is helpful. If the anion gap ([plasma sodium + potassium] – [plasma chloride + bicarbonate]) is >18 mmol/l, this suggests lactic acidosis. A blood lactate concentration >5 mmol/l confirms the diagnosis.

ACUTE CIRCULATORY DISEASE AND DIABETES

Circulatory disease (predominantly coronary heart disease, peripheral vascular disease, and cerebral disease) is three times as common in diabetes sufferers than in those without diabetes. In addition to managing these complications appropriately when they occur it is vital to address individual risk factors in order to prevent these complications. These topics are discussed in detail within Chapter 3 of this book.

DIABETES AND SURGERY – PERIOPERATIVE CONSIDERATIONS

Diabetic patients undergoing surgery are at increased risk compared with nondiabetic patients. There is evidence that both morbidity and mortality rates are increased. Surgical risk is increased in the presence of microvascular, macrovascular, and cardiac complications. Perioperative care of the patient with diabetes should aim to avoid derangement of blood glucose, electrolytes, and fluid balance and prevent the development of a catabolic state.

Hypoglycaemia should be avoided during surgery since it may be difficult to detect. There is evidence, however, that a high glucose concentration (>14 mmol/l) may delay tissue healing, increases ischaemic damage to myocardium and brain, and increases the incidence of surgical infection.

Unless unavoidable, surgery should not commence in patients who are hypoglycaemic or significantly hyperglycaemic. Patients should be starved for at least 4 hours prior to surgery and clear fluids avoided for 2 hours prior to surgery. A less aggressive approach to preoperative starvation reduces the risk of lipolysis, protein catabolism, and loss of electrolytes. However, where gastroparesis may be present the period of starvation should be lengthened to reduce the risk of aspiration. Antiemetics should be used liberally to prevent pre- and postoperative nausea and vomiting.

The catabolic stress of surgery tends to lead to hyperglycaemia with increased release of stress hormones and increased insulin resistance. Early mobility postoperatively reduces the risk of hyperglycaemia.

A preoperative assessment should include a detailed history and examination including the following information:
❑ Type of diabetes.
❑ Duration of diabetes.
❑ Current treatment.
❑ Ischaemic heart disease.
❑ Cardiac failure.
❑ Hypertension.
❑ Renal disease.
❑ Glucose control.
❑ Foot disease.
❑ Autonomic neuropathy.
❑ Eye disease.
❑ Presence of cheiroarthropathy.
❑ Lung disease.
Investigations prior to surgery should include:
❑ Plasma glucose.
❑ Urea and electrolytes.
❑ Full blood count.
❑ Urinalysis.
❑ Echocardiogram.
❑ Additional tests that are appropriate for the procedure.

LONG-TERM COMPLICATIONS
DIABETIC RETINOPATHY
Retinopathy is a common microvascular complication in patients with Type 1 and Type 2 diabetes.

In the UK, diabetes remains the leading cause of blindness for those below the age of 60 years. Retinopathy is strongly associated with duration of diabetes and is more common in those with poor glycaemic control. It is also more common in men and where there are other microvascular complications of diabetes and in hypertension.

In Type 1 diabetes, significant retinopathy is uncommon in the first 5 years after diagnosis. At 10 years, 50% of patients have at least background retinopathy and at 20 years nearly all have at least background retinopathy. In Type 2 diabetes, about 20% will have retinopathy at diagnosis. Most will have a degree of retinopathy after 20 years of diagnosis. Retinopathy is commonest in older people and those treated with insulin. Maculopathy is particularly prevalent in people with Type 2 diabetes, occurring in 25% of those with Type 2 diabetes of 20 years duration. It is the leading cause of blindness in this group.

Although good glycaemic control is associated with a lower risk of developing diabetic retinopathy, intensified glucose control can lead to a worsening of retinopathy in the first year after control is improved. This may relate to a reduction in blood flow that worsens the ischaemic damage. The long-term benefit of good glycaemic control outweighs any short-term deterioration. Strict blood glucose and blood pressure control has been shown to reduce the risk of developing or worsening diabetic retinopathy. There is evidence that the angiotensin-converting enzyme (ACE) inhibitors also reduce progression in normotensive patients.

Pregnancy is associated with a worsening of retinopathy. Pregnant patients with retinopathy should receive monthly retinal review. Patients with proliferative retinopathy require urgent referral for laser photocoagulation. Those with proliferative retinopathy or progressive ischaemic disease should delay pregnancy until treated.

The stages of diabetic retinopathy
The features of diabetic retinopathy can be observed by direct opthalmoscopy in a darkened room through dilated pupils, through an indirect slit-lamp technique, or via digital fundus photography. A normal fundus is shown in figure **12**.

Diabetic retinopathy can be classified into four categories: background, preproliferative, proliferative, and maculopathy.

Background retinopathy is characterized by the presence of one or more of the following (**13**):

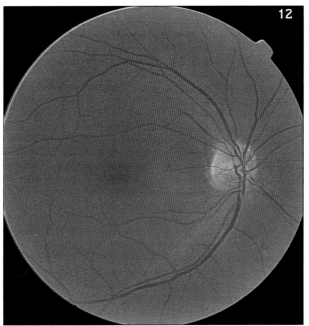

12 A normal fundus.

13 Background retinopathy.

❏ Microaneurysms. These are outgrowths of retinal capillaries, developing from weakening of capillary walls. These are typically the first detectable signs of retinopathy. They appear as small red dots and vary in size from 20–200 μm. They can appear and disappear and occur most commonly at the pole of the eye and in the temporal region adjacent to the macula.

❏ Intraretinal haemorrhages. If occurring deep in the retina, these lesions give the appearance of 'blots'. Larger blots are associated with retinal ischaemia. More superficial haemorrhages are flame-shaped and typically are associated with hypertension.

❏ Hard exudates. These are lipoprotein deposits leaked from capillaries. They are yellowish-white in appearance with a waxy appearance. They appear as dots, streaks or 'circinate' rings. Circinate exudates surround a focal area of leaking vessels.

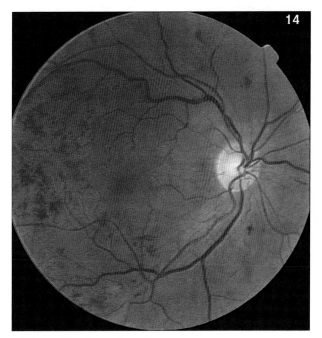

14 Preproliferative retinopathy.

Preproliferative retinopathy (**14**) is characterized by the presence of the following (typically in combination with features of background retinopathy):

❏ Venous beading. These are characteristic changes in the appearance of retinal veins where segmental dilatations give the appearance of a 'string of sausages'. Venous beading suggest severe retinal ischaemia and is associated with an increased risk of new vessel formation. Venous 'loops' may also be seen.

❏ Intravascular microvascular abnormalities (IRMAs). These are capillaries of abnormal appearance. They form a lacy network within the retina and are a sign of retinal ischaemia. They are associated with a high risk of new vessel formation.

❏ Cottonwool spots. These are retinal infarcts that appear as blurred rounded lesions in the nerve fibre layer. They are found most commonly in the nasal side and mid-periphery close to visible vessels. When found in abundance they are associated with a high risk for the development of proliferative retinopathy. More than five cottonwool spots is indicative of preproliferative retinopathy.

❏ Arterial changes. In diabetic retinopathy, arterioles can become tortuous and narrowed. When completely occluded, a white line may be left in place of the arteriole. This is indicative of retinal ischaemia.

Proliferative retinopathy (15) is an urgent sight-threatening complication characterized by new retinal blood vessel formation. It is characterized by:

❏ New vessel formation (neovascularization). These are indicative of proliferative retinopathy. They develop in response to growth factors from the ischaemic retina (vascular endothelium-derived growth factor [VEGF]). New vessels are very fine and branching. They grow from intraretinal veins that lie within the retina and extend through the internal limiting membrane that lines the retina. They tend to grow on the optic disc or the mid-periphery of the retina. New vessels on the disc carry the highest risk of progression to visual loss. When new vessels grow on the iris, this is termed rubeosis iridis. This can obstruct drainage channels for the aqueous and lead to glaucoma.

❏ Preretinal haemorrhages. These occur as a result of bleeding from new vessels. They form a flat-topped (boat-shaped) appearance on fundoscopy.

❏ Vitreous haemorrhage. This is a serious complication of new vessel formation. Dense vitreous haemorrhage causes visual loss. It appears as a dark opacity on fundoscopy and obscures visualization of the retina.

❏ Fibrous bands. These are white/grey scar tissue, frequently seen around blood vessel arcades in proliferative disease. These scars can contract and cause traction retinal detachment and accompanying visual loss.

Maculopathy (16) results from retinal oedema occurring within one optic disc diameter of the macula. Hard exudates, including circinate rings are common and may surround the macula. Maculopathy can lead to severe loss of central vision.

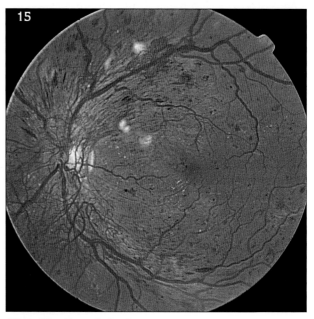

15 Proliferative retinopathy.

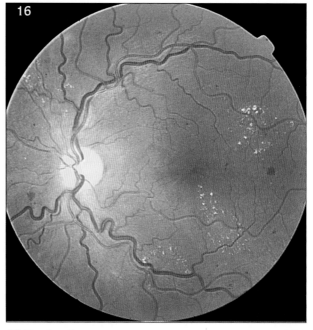

16 Maculopathy.

Complications of laser treatment (**17**) include pain, temporary visual loss, reduced visual acuity, and reduced visual field loss. This may affect government requirements for obtaining a driving license. Surgical vitrectomy may be necessary where there is persistent vitreous haemorrhage with recent retinal detachment (**18**). The vitreous is removed and replaced with saline. Fibrous membranes can be dissected to reduce the risk of further detachment. This procedure can be accompanied by laser photocoagulation. In experienced hands, the majority get a successful result from surgery. A recently detached retina can also be replaced and recent retinal tears can be repaired. Neovascular glaucoma secondary to rubeosis iridis can cause acute painful loss of vision and sometimes enucleation may be the only effective treatment.

Screening for diabetic retinopathy

Diabetic retinopathy is initially symptom-free and retinal screening is an essential component of a diabetes care plan. In Type 1 diabetes, sight-threatening retinopathy is rare before 5 years from diagnosis. After 5 years, however, annual screening should be performed. In Type 2 diabetes screening should be at diagnosis and annually thereafter.

Where there is high risk for the development of sight-threatening retinopathy the screening duration should be increased to every 3–6 months. This includes where there is rapid improvements in blood glucose control, during pregnancy, severe hypertension, or where nephropathy is present. Significant retinopathy also warrants early review. This includes new or worsening retinal changes and scattered exudates less than 1 disc diameter from the fovea.

Screening for diabetic retinopathy should include an assessment of visual acuity with glasses or through a pinhole. This can be done with a Snellen chart from 6 metres. Eye examination should be carried out by retinal photography, conducted and evaluated by trained personnel or by slit-lamp indirect opthalmoscopy in trained hands. Unless contra-indicated, tropicamide should be used to dilate pupils.

> *The National Service Framework for Diabetes specifies that digital retinal photography is the method of choice for retinopathy screening. It is expected that all diabetic patients should be receiving annual retinal screening by the end of 2007. The establishment of national retinal screening audit standards and a national retinal screening register is accompanying this initiative. However, this has not yet happened.*

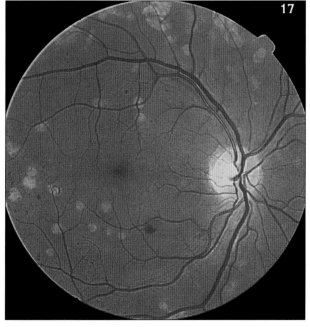

17 Laser photocoagulation.

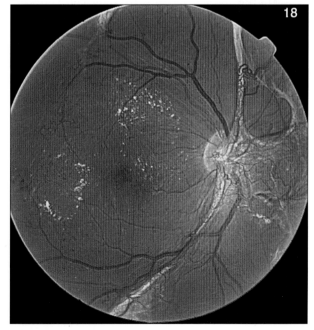

18 Retinal detachment.

Patients with sudden loss of vision or evidence of retinal detachment should be seen by an ophthalmologist immediately. Those with new vessel formation, evidence of vitreous or preretinal haemorrhage, or rubeosis iridis should be seen within 1 week. If there is an unexplained drop in visual acuity, hard exudates within one disc diameter of the fovea, macular oedema, unexplained retinal findings, or preproliferative/severe retinopathy, the patient should be seen within 4 weeks.

OTHER EYE COMPLICATIONS
Cataract
Cataracts are more common in diabetes. They also develop earlier and progress more quickly. Hyperglycaemia causes nonenzymatic glycation of lens proteins. The most common is a cortical cataract that gives a 'spokewheel' appearance on ophthalmoscopy. Central lens opacification ultimately leads to loss of vision. Other forms include a posterior subcapsular cataract that causes early visual loss and a snowflake cataract that occurs rapidly in younger people but can clear spontaneously.

Ocular nerve palsies
Diabetes can cause a nerve palsy of the third or sixth nerve. This leads to sudden onset of painless diplopia. Typically, but not in all cases, the condition resolves slowly over the course of several weeks or months. With third nerve palsy it is important to exclude an intracranial aneurysm and it may be wise to investigate these patients with magnetic resonance imaging (MRI).

Sudden loss of vision
Vitreous hamorrhage is a common cause of sudden visual loss in patients with diabetes but other conditions should be considered. Retinal detachment presents as flashes and floaters with a grey curtain in the periphery of vision. Urgent re-attachment of the retina with laser or cryotherapy may restore vision if undertaken within a day or two of the event.

Central retinal vein occlusion as a cause of sudden visual loss is more common in diabetes, particularly where there is co-existent hypertension. Vision may be moderately or severely affected. Ophthalmoscopy reveals disc oedema and widespread retinal haemorrhages. In 10% of sufferers, the second eye will subsequently develop the same problem. In the affected eye there is a high risk of retinal ischaemia with subsequent new vessel formation. Regular retinal

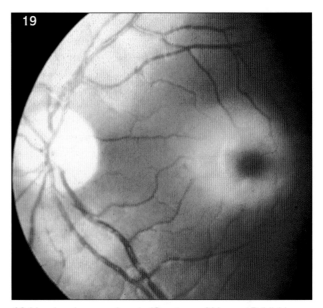

19 Macular cherry red spot. (Courtesy of Manson Publishing: *Paediatrics and Child Health*, 2007.)

review is therefore essential. Branch vein occlusions may occur, restricting the abnormalities to just one quadrant.

Central retinal artery occlusion causes painless loss of vision. It is more common in older patients (>60 years). The cause is retinal artery thrombosis or embolism. There may be a preceding history of transient visual loss from one eye (amaurosis fugax). Ophthalmoscopy may be unremarkable in the early stages but pallor develops with 'threadlike' arterioles and a prominent fovea (cherry red spot [**19**]). The visual loss is permanent and may be severe if the macula is involved. The patient should be assessed to exclude cardiac disease, carotid disease, hypertension, hyperlipidaemia, and temporal arteritis.

Ischaemic optic neuropathy can lead to infarction of the optic disc and sudden onset of central visual loss. Ophthalmoscopy reveals a pale swollen disc with flame-shaped haemorrhages.

NEPHROPATHY AND RENAL DISEASE
Diabetic nephropathy is one of the commonest causes of end-stage renal failure. It accounts for one-third of all UK patients accepted for dialysis treatment. In Type 1 diabetes, patients diagnosed at a young age (<30 years) are at greatest risk. The prevalence of diabetic nephropathy increases with

duration of diabetes. At 30 years, about 1 in 3 patients with Type 1 diabetes will have evidence of nephropathy. This suggests that some are protected. The risk of progressing to end-stage renal failure is greatly lessened with tight glycaemic control. Those with the worst glucose control have a fourfold greater risk than those with the best control. Asian and Afro-Caribbean populations have a greater risk of nephropathy.

Although it is less likely in Type 2 diabetes, the explosion of Type 2 diabetes prevalence means that Type 2 diabetes is now a more common cause of nephropathy than Type 1 diabetes.

Diabetic nephropathy is characterized by increased protein loss in the urine. Protein leakage is caused by an increase in transglomerular pressure. A loss of negative charge on the basement membrane and epithelial cell foot processes occurs. This reduces the repulsion between the membrane and albumin molecules. Larger pores develop and ultimately tubular damage occurs. Kidney glomeruli become enlarged early in diabetes. Thickening of the basement membrane and expansion of the mesangium that supports tufts of capillaries cause this. There are also renal tubular changes that include basement membrane thickening, interstitial fibrosis, arteriosclerosis, and atrophy. Nodules may form within glomeruli, leading to the characteristic 'Kimmelstiel–Wilson' appearance of nodular glomerulosclerosis.

Glomerular filtration rate (GFR) increases initially in early diabetic nephropathy but then declines as glomeruli become occluded. Microalbuminuria is the first obvious clinical development. This can be ascertained from an early morning urine sample. The test is a urine albumin:creatinine ratio (ACR). If the ACR is greater than 2.5 mg/mmol in men or 3.5 mg/mmol in women, this is suggestive of microalbuminuria.

Dip-stick-positive proteinuria (Albustix) occurs when 24 hour urinary levels exceed 300 mg. This is approximately ten times the level at which micro-albuminuria is detected by immunoassay.

A daily urinary albumin loss of more than 3.5 g can be a later dvelopment and is characteristic of the nephrotic syndrome.

As renal glomeruli gradually sclerose, the remaining glomeruli face further increases in blood flow and nephrons fail. When a critical number of nephrons are lost, the GFR starts to drop dramatically and this leads to progressive renal failure (20). Co-existent hypertension accelerates this process.

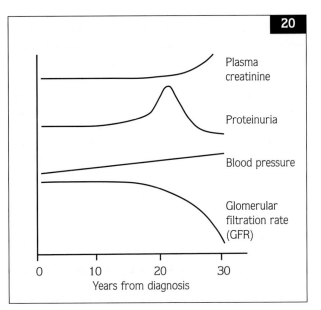

20 Diagram to show the natural history of diabetic nephropathy.

Screening for diabetic nephropathy

An annual early morning urinary albumin:creatinine ratio should be performed to detect the presence of microalbuminuria. If elevated this should be repeated twice.

When proteinuria is present in the absence of retinopathy (which usually precedes the development of nephropathy) or where there is a short duration of Type 1 diabetes (<5 years), diagnoses other than diabetic nephropathy should be considered. Other investigations should then include urine culture and microscopy (for red cells and casts), serum markers for connective tissue disease (rheumatoid factor, complement levels, and anti-DNA antibodies), a myeloma screen, and a renal ultrasound scan. Where doubt remains, a renal biopsy should be performed.

Other renal complications of diabetes

Both hypertensive renal disease and vascular renal disease are more common in diabetes. They frequently co-exist with diabetic nephropathy in patients with diabetic renal disease.

Renal artery stenosis (RAS) is an important disorder associated with hypertension and worsening renal function. RAS is more common in diabetes than in the general population. It is particularly common in Type 2 diabetes, affecting about 1 in 12 patients.

It is strongly associated with the presence of peripheral vascular disease. In RAS, audible bruits may be heard over the site of the stenosis. It may present with sudden onset of pulmonary oedema.

In unilateral disease, a renal ultrasound scan may show asymmetrical kidney size. Colour flow Doppler studies provide a superior noninvasive investigation but arteriography is the gold standard technique for identifying the site of lesions. Urinary tract infections and pyelonephritis are more common in diabetes. There is a wide range of pathogenic bacteria. Candidal vaginitis or balanitis is a common presentation of diabetes. Bladder outflow obstruction due to autonomic neuropathy is more common in diabetes.

DIABETIC NEUROPATHY AND FOOT DISEASE

Diabetes can affect both central and peripheral nerves but the term tends to be used to describe disease of the peripheral nerves. There are several different forms of diabetic neuropathy:
- ❏ Sensorimotor neuropathy.
- ❏ Proximal motor neuropathy.
- ❏ Mononeuropathies.
- ❏ Autonomic neuropathy.

Chronic sensorimotor neuropathy is present in up to 60% of patients with diabetes although abnormalities on history and examination are found in only 20%.

The mechanism is not fully understood but there are clear links with the impairment of blood supply to myelinated and unmyelinated nerve fibres. Nerve damage may be sporadic and nonselective with a predilection for the longest nerves, principally those supplying the feet, and to a lesser extent, the hands. This gives the characteristic 'glove and stocking' distribution of sensory loss.

Patients with this condition are at increased risk of developing retinopathy and nephropathy. The development of diabetic neuropathy is known to be associated most strongly with increased duration of diabetes and poor glucose control.

Risk factors for the development of sensorimotor neuropathy include:
- ❏ Increased age.
- ❏ Poor glycaemic control.
- ❏ Increased duration of diabetes.
- ❏ Smoking.
- ❏ Other microvascular complications (nephropathy, retinopathy).
- ❏ Dyslipidaemia (low levels of high-density lipoprotein [HDL]-cholesterol).

In patients where neuropathy is suspected, there should be specific questioning about the presence of back pain and bowel/bladder function. It is essential to rule out other causes of foot/leg pain and the other causes of peripheral neuropathy (*Table 10*).

It is essential when assessing a patient with a foot condition to take a detailed history of the type, frequency, and nature of any pain, tenderness, paraesthesia, or numbness. In addition, any precipitating and alleviating factors and associated symptoms should be recorded.

Neuropathic pain may be severe and it is important to allow the patient to express their feelings and for the listener to be empathetic. The pain itself may be variably described as shooting, stabbing, burning, aching, tender, strange. An assessment of the impact of symptoms should be made. The pain can be worse at night, keeping the patient awake. Patients may not be able to bear the touch of the sheets against the skin and may resort to hanging feet over the edge of the bed.

A full physical examination should be carried out. This should include a clinical neurological assessment. Pain is subjective and it may be important to identify tools that enable symptoms to be quantified. Pain questionnaires are used widely to assist in the detection and severity of pain and in the evaluation of treatment. Tools used for the assessment and detection of neuropathy can be simple. These include the assessment of ankle/knee reflexes using a tendon hammer, assessment of vibration perception with the use of a 128 Hz tuning fork, light touch/pressure sensation using a cotton-

Table 10 Causes of peripheral neuropathy	
Metabolic	Diabetes, uraemia, amyloidosis, myxoedema, and porphyria
Nutritional	B12, B6, nicotinic acid, or thiamine deficiencies
Drug/chemical	Nitrofurantoin, vincristine, chloambucil, isoniazid, phenytoin
Neoplasia	Bronchogenic carcinoma, malignant lymphoma
Infection	Guillain–Barré syndrome, leprosy
Genetic	Charcot–Marie–Tooth syndrome
Organ failure	Renal and hepatic failure

wool swab or 10 g monofilament, and pain sensation using the 'Neurotip' or a neurological pin. Decreased vibration sense and absent ankle jerks are the earliest signs of diabetic neuropathy. Loss of sensation is most marked distally.

Other neuropathies associated with diabetes

Diabetic amyotrophy

This condition presents with severe pain, tenderness and paraesthesiae in the upper legs. It is associated with weakness and wasting of the quadriceps muscles. Weight loss may be an accompanying feature or the only symptom. Examination reveals wasting of the quadriceps, tenderness of the anterior thigh, and reduced hip flexion power. Knee jerks may be absent. The condition may be asymmetrical. The condition occurs as a result of damage to the lower motor neurones of the lumbosacral plexus. It affects older patients and may be associated with poor glucose control. The condition should be self-limiting, lasting a few weeks or months.

Mononeuropathies

Spontaneous diabetic mononeuropathies are acute, suggesting a vascular cause. The cranial nerves (third and sixth (see page 32), fourth, and seventh) are most frequently affected. Entrapment nerve palsies are more common in diabetes. Carpal tunnel syndrome affecting the median nerve at the wrist may affect up to 10% of diabetic patients. Another affected nerve is the lateral cutaneous nerve of the thigh at the inguinal ligament. This causes pain and paraesthesia over the lateral aspect of the thigh (meralgia paraesthetica). External pressure palsies affecting the radial, ulnar, and peroneal nerves are more common in diabetes.

Autonomic neuropathy

Diabetic autonomic neuropathy is due to impaired function of the small unmyelinated nerve fibres that help to control the autonomic nervous system. A significant proportion of patients have some degree of autonomic dysfunction on direct testing but most do not experience significant symptoms. It is associated with other microvascular complications and also with sudden death. The frequency of autonomic neuropathy increases with duration of diabetes and is also associated with poor glucose control. Symptomatic autonomic neuropathy is more common in Type 1 diabetes.

There is evidence that diabetic autonomic neuropathy plays a part in the development of erectile dysfunction in diabetic men (see Erectile dysfunction, page 39).

Other symptoms include dizziness and blackouts due to postural hypotension. Nausea, vomiting and diarrhoea occur secondary to gastroparesis. Bladder dysfunction is occasionally a problem. Gustatory sweating is a symptom characterized by facial sweating that occurs during and after eating. Increased sweating over the upper half of the body can also be a distressing symptom.

Physical signs include dry skin, particularly affecting the feet, postural hypotension, tachycardia, absence of sinus arrhythmia, and small pupils.

There are a number of available investigations. These include the heart rate response to standing or deep breathing and the blood pressure response to standing or a sustained handgrip. Variability in heart rate is calculated by calculating the shortest R-R interval on echocardiogram (ECG) inspection during inspiration and the longest R-R interval on expiration. There is less variability in cases of autonomic dysfunction. Postural hypotension is defined by a reduction in systolic blood pressure (2 minutes after standing) of >20 mmHg.

Peripheral vascular disease (PVD) in diabetes

The circulatory disease of the leg seen in diabetes is different to that of the nondiabetic. The involvement is variable. There may be diffuse atherosclerotic changes, patchy distribution, or markedly distal distribution of disease.

Macrovascular disease in the diabetic leg can occur at the iliac, femoral, popliteal, and tibial regions. Those with diabetes have a higher incidence of disease in the arteries distal to the popliteal and have more diffuse vessel involvement. In those with diabetes, atherosclerosis tends to be 'multi-segmental' rather than involving a single region of arterial wall. Arterial calcification is commonly observed in radiographs of diabetic feet and hands. This is due to calcification of the media in muscular arteries. Its importance in determining blood flow is not clear but its effects are probably not significant. Damage to small blood vessels in the feet of diabetic individuals leads to capillary leakage of albumin. Other findings on microscopic examination include obliterative lesions of arterioles and capillaries with basement membrane thickening and endothelial proliferation, but the importance of these findings in determining circulation is not known.

Intermittent claudication and rest pain may be presenting symptoms of major vessel disease. Exercise-induced buttock or calf pain are typical.

Worsening claudication or rest pain indicate more critical ischaemia. On examination of the diabetic foot the absence of pedal and posterior tibial pulses is an important finding since it indicates the presence of macrovascular disease

Minor trauma is often the precipitating factor for tissue damage in the ischaemic foot. Simple trauma includes pressure from ill-fitting shoes or even tight socks. Injuries may originate from the cutting of toenails or thermal and chemical injuries. Secondary infection commonly occurs. In the ischaemic foot there is frequently blockage of the metatarsal arteries and this reduces communication between plantar and dorsal arterial arches. This lack of collateral circulation can be devastating since bacteria may produce toxic products that cause direct damage to local blood vessels.

Those with diabetes have a 16-fold increased risk of amputation and 1 in 5 will die within 2 years of the onset of symptoms. Ischaemic foot ulceration is frequently painful and may only respond to opioid analgesia.

The diabetic foot

People with diabetes and those caring for them should be provided with easy access to a multidisciplinary diabetic foot care team. This should be a team of people who work closely together in settings that allow for easy communication and direct access to each other's specialist skills. Ideally the diabetic team should include the following members:
- Specialist podiatrist.
- Specialist orthotist.
- Diabetes nurse specialist.
- Diabetologist.
- Vascular surgeon.
- Orthopaedic surgeon.

A programme of foot care should be provided to ensure that patients are educated about the prevention of foot disease and that the at-risk or diseased foot can be identified early. There should be links between and within primary and secondary care to ensure that risk factors and complications are managed effectively.

Those with diabetes can suffer a range of foot complications. Foot ulceration is common. In the UK, its prevalence is at least 5%. There are a number of factors associated with the development of diabetic foot ulceration. It is usually caused by a combination of abnormal foot shape with neuropathy and/or impairment of blood supply.

Foot deformities in diabetes

Deformities in the diabetic foot may be due in part to a limitation of joint mobility. There is abnormal glycosylation of connective tissue that in turn leads to a limitation of joint movement and leads to functional foot problems. Foot deformities lead to altered pressure loads within the feet. Localized high-pressure areas are caused by abnormal bony prominences. In the neuropathic foot, elevated local pressure increases the likelihood of developing hyperkeratosis and subsequent callus formation. Callus causes a further elevation in plantar pressure and this can eventually lead to ulceration. Where blood supply to the foot is impaired, excessive pressures can lead directly to foot tissue damage and subsequent ulceration. Normalizing foot function is important in preserving normal plantar pressures during walking.

Hallux rigidus, pes cavus, ankle equinus, and claw or hammer toe are common deformities that can lead to an increase in pressure loads on the plantar surface of the forefoot, metatarsal heads, or tips of the toes and the dorsal surface of interphalangeal joints. Charcot deformities, nail abnormalities, peripheral oedema, and deformities secondary to surgical procedures also increase the risk of foot ulceration. Ulceration can develop when the nail penetrates tissue as a result of ingrowing toenails that are due to excessive convexity of the nail plate or poor nail care. Peripheral oedema is frequently found in patients with diabetes, particularly in the elderly. It may exist as a marker of congestive cardiac failure, more commonly seen in patients with diabetes.

Oedema is sometimes found in patients with severe diabetic neuropathy who have no cardiac disease or other obvious underlying cause. This is due to increased venous pressure resulting from a reduction of sympathetic tone. Oedema is a significant risk factor for the development of foot ulceration and may delay the recovery from preexisting foot ulceration. It results in a tighter shoe fit and therefore increases the pressure effects of ill-fitting shoes.

Digital (Ray) amputation is the commonest procedure carried out for digital gangrene, a complication that occurs as a result of neuropathic or neuro-ischaemic damage to a toe. The amputation is often curative but affects the biomechanics of the foot and increases the risk of further ulceration under metatarsal heads.

Peripheral neuropathy can lead to weakness and wasting of the intrinsic foot muscles with subsequent toe deformities. It also leads to abnormal pressure distribution and the creation of an ill-fitting effect in previous well-fitting footwear. Dryness and fissuring of skin is a frequent feature of diabetic neuropathy, probably as an effect of reduced sweating relating to impaired autonomic function. Cracks in the skin provide an entry site for secondary infection.

Neuropathy and foot ulceration
Neuropathic ulceration is commonly found on the tip of a toe or underneath a metatarsal head. It can also be found on the dorsum of the toe, between toes, or underneath the heel. Its appearance is typically 'punched out' (**21**). The lesion is often circular, particularly on the sole of the foot, and has surrounding callus formation. It is typically painless but may penetrate to involve deeper tissues, including bone. Neuropathic ulceration occurs partly because of a reduction in pain sensation. Loss of pain awareness enables the development and progression of foot lesions to proceed unchecked.

Neglected callus formation can occur as a result of increased vertical and shear forces beneath the metatarsal heads or excessive friction at the tips of the toes as a result of walking and recurrent trauma of toe against footwear. Repetitive friction or pressure leads to cell damage, microscopic haemorrhage, and callus formation. Tissue damage and necrosis beneath callus leads to the development of small cavities that can fill with serous fluid and erupt onto the surface of the foot as an ulcer. Ulceration may also develop from more direct trauma such as treading on sharp objects or from debris and irregular surfaces arising from within footwear.

Some foot ulcers originate from direct heat trauma from placing feet directly in front of fires and radiators, bathing feet in excessively hot water, or against hot water bottles. Loss of pain awareness prevents the sufferer from moving his feet away from these stimuli and direct damage to epithelium then occurs. Chemical burns can similarly occur from using solutions that contain salicylic acid, commonly used for treating warts and corns.

Fungal infections are more common in those with diabetes and occur commonly in the interdigital spaces. This can lead to cracks and breaches in the skin. Secondary infection and ulceration may ensue.

Autonomic and motor neuropathy can also contribute to the development of neuropathic ulceration. Autonomic neuropathy leads to dryness of the skin and can also lead to arterio-venous shunting which may affect the perfusion of skin and bone.

Motor neuropathy contributes to the paralysis of small muscles in the feet that in turn may exacerbate structural abnormalities. The classical example of this is clawing of the toes that leads to prominent metatarsal heads and accompanying high-pressure zones.

Ischaemia and foot ulceration
Ulceration is a common feature of the neuro-ischaemic foot. Typically there is an area of necrosis surrounded by a rim of erythema. The typical sites for ulceration are the great toe, the medial surface of the first metatarsal head, and the heel (**22**). Unlike neuropathic ulceration it is frequently painful.

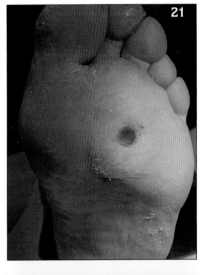

21 Neuropathic ulcer.

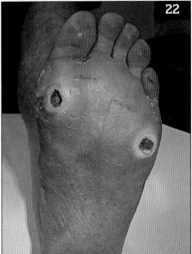

22 The neuroischaemic foot.

Infection and foot ulceration

Secondary infection frequently contributes to the persistence and worsening of foot ulceration (**23**). A range of organisms is involved, including anaerobic organisms, Gram-negative bacilli, cocci, and gas-forming organisms Clostridia, *E. coli* and *Bacteroides* sp. Spreading cellulitis can develop in surrounding skin or in deeper tissues. Tendons, joints, and bones can also become infected. Bacteria and toxins may invade systemically to cause a bacteraemia. Other complications of infection include local necrosis and gangrene (**24, 25**). These can result from damage to microcirculation even when major foot pulses are present.

The prevention of diabetic foot disease

The avoidance of foot ulceration is an important aspect in the management of patients with diabetes. Foot ulceration places a patient at high risk of subsequent amputation.

This can be helped by recommending appropriate footwear and foot care advice to patients with diabetes, in particular those at high risk of foot ulceration.

Daily inspection of the feet by the patient or a partner enables the early detection of callus and skin lesions that may not be felt by the sufferer. Regular lubrication of dry feet with a simple emollient such as E45 cream reduces the risk of cracks in the skin leading to secondary infection. The provision of appropriate well-fitted footwear with appropriate toe

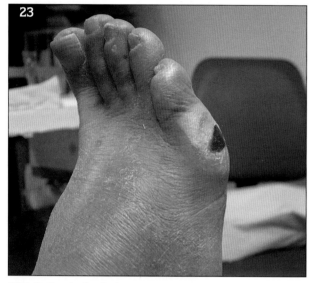

23 Infection in the foot.

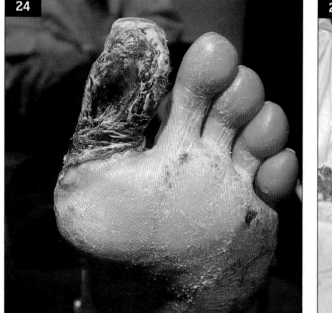

24 Gangrene in the foot.

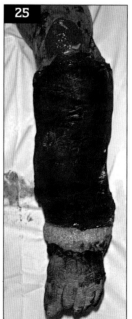

25 Widespread gangrene.

depth and soft uppers is vital. A trained practitioner should care for the toenails of patients at high risk of foot ulceration. Any foot lesions should be inspected and appropriately treated soon after identification. All patients should receive an annual foot assessment to identify those at high risk of foot ulceration. This should form part of an annual diabetes review.

Charcot foot

Charcot foot (neuro-arthropathy) occurs in those with peripheral neuropathy and a good vascular supply. It can occur in patients with both Type 1 and Type 2 diabetes.

Bone damage coincides with an increase in blood flow that may be secondary to the loss of sympathetic nerve supply associated with neuropathic disease. This causes increased osteoclast activity within bone and bone turnover is increased. Bone becomes more prone to damage and fracture from minor trauma and there is subsequent destruction of bony architecture. This problem is compounded by peripheral neuropathy that leads to an altered gait pattern and a reduced range of joint motion. The patient frequently presents with a hot, swollen foot that may be painful. Additional complaints include odd creaking noises in the feet and uncomfortable sensations. The typical affected site is the tarsal–metatarsal region or the metatarso-phalangeal joints.

In the Charcot foot peripheral pulses are invariably present and peripheral neuropathy is evident clinically. The affected foot is usually warm.

Trauma may be the trigger for the development of Charcot foot but in the neuropathic patient this may pass unnoticed. The differential diagnoses for acute Charcot disease include cellulitis, gout, and deep vein thrombosis. Radiographic imaging and isotope bone scans can assist in diagnosis.

As the disease progresses the structure of the foot is destroyed. Joint dislocations and fractures occur. These are often in the mid-foot, leading to the collapse of the arch. This can result in a rocker-bottom deformity, due to displacement and subluxation of the tarsus or medial convexity due to the talo-navicular joint or tarso-metatarsal dislocation (26). Figure 27 shows an ulcer overlying a Charcot foot deformity.

ERECTILE DYSFUNCTION

Erectile dysfunction (ED) or impotence is the inability to achieve or maintain an erection sufficient for sexual intercourse. It is both common and distressing and is present in at least one-third of diabetic males. Its prevalence relates strongly to age with over half of

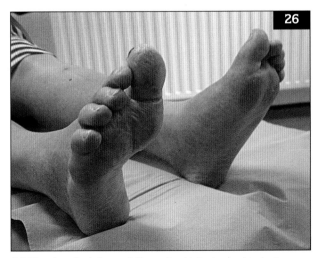

26 The chronic deformed Charcot mid-foot – rocker-bottom deformity.

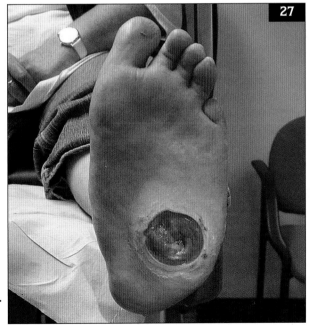

27 The ulcerated Charcot foot.

diabetic males over the age of 55 years suffering with this condition. Other risk factors for the development of ED are excessive alcohol intake, poor glucose control, peripheral vascular disease, and microvascular disease.

Common causes of erectile dysfunction include psychological disease, local vascular disease (arterial insufficiency or venous leaks), endocrine disease (hypothyroidism, hypogonadism and hyperprolactinaemia), neurological disease (peripheral or autonomic neuropathy and spinal cord lesions), drug and alcohol-related disease, renal failure, or local anatomical problems. Significant vascular disease occurs in 70% of diabetic patients with ED. Neuropathy plays a part in about 50%. Drugs and psychiatric disease contribute about 15%.

A careful history, examination, and simple biochemical tests help to elucidate the causes of ED. Where possible, the consultation should include the patient and his partner. A thorough history should first clarify the precise nature of the problem since the term 'impotence' may have a different meaning to the patient. The speed of onset should be noted since psychological ED is typically acute. The presence of morning or spontaneous erections also implies a psychological cause.

A medical history should focus on neurological, vascular, and drug history. Symptoms that suggest peripheral or autonomic nerve dysfunction (loss of foot sensation, neuropathic pain, gastroparesis, and postural hypotension) are helpful in suggesting a neuropathic aetiology. Bladder dysfunction or a history of central nervous system disease can indicate a spinal or brain lesion. A history of ischaemic heart disease, peripheral vascular disease, raised blood pressure, smoking, and dyslipidaemia can suggest a vascular cause. The presence of renal disease and retinopathy should be noted. Symptoms suggestive of endocrine disease may be present (reduced libido, tiredness, and loss of body hair).

Ill health and hyperglycaemia can contribute to transient ED and should be enquired about. It may be helpful to ascertain whether there are relationship difficulties, anxieties, stress, and loss of self-esteem. A drug history should focus on antihypertensive therapies, antidepressants, antipsychotics, diuretics, and alcohol as potential causes. The timing of symptoms in relation to the start of drug therapy should be ascertained. Physical examination should include an inspection of the external genitalia for penile and testicular abnormalities. There are a number of possible local causes:

❑ Peyronie's disease.
❑ Phimosis.
❑ Balanitis.
❑ Tumour.
❑ Congenital deformity.
❑ Local penile trauma.
❑ Absent, shrunken, or diseased testes.

The patient should also be examined for the presence of secondary sexual characteristics. A cardiovascular and neurological examination should be performed.

> *Baseline laboratory investigations for ED should include an HbA1c, serum creatinine, thyroid function, serum prolactin, and testosterone.*

Further investigations are rarely required. A detailed psychosexual assessment will be necessary for some. A penile Doppler ultrasound scan may give an idea of the degree of blood supply impairment and can be followed up with arteriography of the internal iliac vessels. Cavernosography may be helpful in those who fail to respond to therapy. This involves the rapid infusion of saline into the corpus cavernosum followed by the injection of contrast medium. It can be used to detect venous leaks.

The measurement of nocturnal penile rigidity using a penile strain gauge can help to differentiate between physical and psychological ED. The strain gauge is connected to a recording device and measures penile circumference overnight.

GASTROINTESTINAL CONDITIONS ASSOCIATED WITH DIABETES

Complications of diabetes affecting the gastrointestinal tract are uncommon but can be distressing and difficult to treat. They are summarized in *Table 11*.

SKIN DISEASE

A range of skin conditions can be associated with diabetes. These are typically benign but can be unsightly, irritating or upsetting for patients.

Diabetic dermopathy

This is the most commonly seen skin condition. It presents with small rounded papules, reddish in colour. They occur in clusters and are commonly seen in older patients. They tend to atrophy and scar over a period of years. They tend to be found on limbs, particularly the shins and forearms. There is no effective treatment.

Table 11 Gastrointestinal conditions associated with diabetes

Site of lesion	Problem	Nature of problem
Whole tract	Candidiasis	Common in diabetes. Affects oral cavity, oesophagus and, rarely, the colon. May require endoscopic diagnosis. Usually treated with nystatin suspension
Oesophagus	Dysphagia	Oesophageal motor disorders and diffuse oesophageal spasm are more common in diabetes. This may be painful. Nitrates, calcium channel blockers, or anticholinergic drugs may help. Occasionally requires surgical myotomy
Stomach	Gastroparesis	Presents with nausea, discomfort, heartburn, and vomiting. Due to reduced gastic emptying. Fatty foods should be avoided. Metoclopramide and domperidone most frequently helpful
Small intestine	Coeliac disease	Found in 3–4% of people with diabetes. Screening for this condition is with gut antibodies (e.g. transglutaminase or antiendomysium antibodies). Definitive diagnosis is by duodenal or jejunal biopsy. It is a cause of malabsorption and is treated by a gluten-free diet
	Chronic pancreatitis	Diabetes may present as a complication of chronic pancreatitis. There is usually associated malabsorption due to inadequate digestive enzymes. Treated with pancreatic enzyme supplements
Large intestine	Diarrhoea	Autonomic neuropathy and bacterial overgrowth can contribute to this in diabetes. There is characteristically passing of a high-volume stool. Neuropathic dysmotility may respond to loperamide or codeine phosphate. Somatostatin analogues have been shown to be useful in some. Bulking agents and antispasmodics may help. Bacterial overgrowth requires a course of metronidazole or tetracycline
Liver	Fatty liver	Particularly common in Type 2 diabetes. Fatty droplets seen within hepatocytes. Characteristic appearance on ultrasound. This is associated with an elevated alkaline phosphatase (20–50% increased) and transaminases at the upper end of normal. This is reduced with weight loss and reduced fat ingestion. Exacerbated by alcohol

Necrobiosis lipoidica

This is typically seen in younger patients, more commonly women with diabetes. The usual site is the shin (28) but it can be seen elsewhere, particularly arms and legs. It is an irregularly-shaped reddish lesion with a central yellow atrophied area and a waxy appearance. The atrophied centre can ulcerate in some individuals. It is caused by collagen degeneration in the dermis. Local steroid injections may be helpful in encouraging healing.

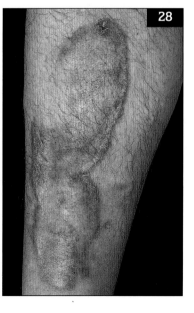

28 Necrobiosis lipoidica. (Courtesy of Manson Publishing: *A Colour Handbook of Dermatology*, 2005.)

Acanthosis nigricans

This is a hyperpigmented epidermal overgrowth with a velvety appearance. It occurs in flexural areas, typically in the axilla (3). It is seen in Type 2 diabetes and as part of the insulin resistance syndrome. It is probably caused by circulating insulin acting on IGF-1 receptors in the skin to stimulate growth.

Cheiroarthropathy

This is a thickening of the skin in diabetes. Excessive glycation of collagen within the dermis leads to limited joint mobility and tight, waxy skin. The 'prayer sign', in which the patient cannot oppose the palmar surfaces of two hands, is used as part of some foot assessment tools. It highlights limitation in joint mobility that can lead to abnormal pressure loads in the feet with an increased risk of ulceration.

Trigger finger, frozen shoulder, and Dupuytren's contracture

These conditions relate to a thickening and fibrosis of the tendon sheath or articular capsule and are more common where there is cheiroathropathy. Steroid injections may help but surgery may be necessary where this is ineffective.

Infective skin and nail conditions

These are more common in diabetes. The most frequent include chronic paronychia, candidal vaginitis/balanitis, and skin boils/pustules secondary to bacterial infections. Topical antifungal agents are helpful for *Candida* and other fungal infections but chronic fungal paronychia may require systemic imidazole therapy.

Lipoatrophy and lipohypertrophy

These are specifically associated with insulin administration.

PSYCHOLOGICAL DISORDERS AND DIABETES

The diagnosis of diabetes has an emotional impact on most patients and their families.

The emotional and psychological response to the diagnosis is dependent upon a range of factors. These include the implications for employment, social activities, and lifestyle. They will depend upon the age of the patient, the treatment required, co-morbid ill health or complications, and the degree of social support or isolation.

The ability of a patient to come to terms with the diagnosis will also depend upon psychological and social factors unique to that individual. This includes their occupation, intelligence, temperament, culture, beliefs, and psychological state.

Emotional effects may include fear of blindness or amputation. Restrictions on daily activity may occur due to insulin administration, blood glucose checking, or concern about glucose levels or hypoglycaemia.

For some, the restrictions on daily life as a result of developing diabetes will be significant and for others the fear of complications will be overwhelming. The impact of diabetes on quality of life for the patient varies according to the individual. This impact may also affect the success of educational programmes. It is therefore important that the approach to diabetes management is individualized. Temporary significant psychological upset is seen in about 30% of children newly diagnosed with diabetes. Symptoms include insomnia, social withdrawal, anxiety, and depression. However this is usually self-limiting. Anxiety states are known to be more common in diabetes than in the general population. Emotional symptoms include fear, nervousness, unease, and panic. Physical symptoms include sweats, shakiness, insomnia, breathlessness, palpitations, numbness and tingling, light-headedness, nausea, and a dry mouth. This can lead to safety-seeking behaviour and isolation.

A common specific fear is hypoglycaemia. This can lead patients to err on the side of hyperglycaemia or develop erratic glucose control due to effects of counter-regulatory stress hormones. Needle phobia can be an issue for many. This may lead to similar disruption of glycaemia control even if the patient is able to self-inject. This can be eased by the use of needle-covers or needle-free devices.

Specific anxieties should be freely but sympathetically discussed with patients.

Depressive illness is twice as common in diabetes compared with the general population. It is more common in patients with micro- and macrovascular complications and in patients who are hospitalized. Typical features of depression can be difficult to identify alongside those of diabetes. Depressive symptoms include:

❏ Low mood.
❏ Tearfulness.
❏ Reduced interest in life activities.
❏ Lack of self-confidence or self-esteem.
❏ Social isolation.
❏ Insomnia (typically early morning wakening or interrupted sleep).

❏ Tiredness.
❏ Lack of energy.
❏ Reduced libido.
❏ Poor concentration.
❏ Slowness of thought.
❏ Feelings of guilt or hopelessness.
❏ Suicidal inclination.
❏ Anxiety or irritability.

Depressive illness has not been shown to relate strongly to glycaemic control. However, for patients with poor glycaemic control, cognitive behavioural therapy delivered by a trained professional has been shown to be effective in lowering HbA1c.

When identified, depression should be managed conventionally with psychological and pharmaceutical measures. Diabetes poses no contraindication to antidepressant medication. For those with psychological problems there should be easy access to mental health professionals.

MACROVASCULAR DISEASE

Circulatory disease is 2–4 times higher in patients with both Type 1 and Type 2 diabetes compared with that of the nondiabetic population. This includes coronary heart disease, stroke, and peripheral vascular disease. Males and females are affected and women lose their premenopausal protection from cardiovascular disease.

Cardiovascular disease is responsible for three-quarters of deaths in those with Type 2 diabetes. The risk of cardiovascular disease in diabetic patients with no previous history of coronary problems is equal to that of nondiabetic patients who have already sustained a myocardial infarction. The combination of Type 1 or Type 2 diabetes with proteinuria increases the risk of mortality from coronary disease dramatically.

Atherosclerotic disease develops sooner and faster in patients with diabetes. Distal coronary and peripheral vessels tend to be affected. There is endothelial dysfunction in the vessels of those with diabetes. There is reduced vasodilatation from nitric oxide-dependent and independent mechanisms. There is increased macrophage and platelet attachment to the endothelium and increased endothelial permeability to fatty products. There are increased advanced glycation end products (AGEs) that lead to increased adhesiveness, procoagulation, and foam cell formation that initiate atheromatous plaque.

The effects of smoking, hypertension and dyslipidaemia on cardiovascular risk are amplified in the presence of diabetes. The mortality rate of diabetic individuals who are significantly hypertensive (>160 mmHg systolic) or who have a significantly elevated cholesterol (>7 mmol/l) is about 80% at 10 years. It has yet to be established whether glucose control has a significant effect on the risk for cardiovascular disease.

Risk factors for atherosclerosis cluster with insulin resistance in the metabolic syndrome. Features of the metabolic syndrome include:
❏ Central obesity.
❏ Hypertension.
❏ Dyslipidaemia (raised triglycerides, reduced HDL-cholesterol).
❏ Elevated insulin levels (associated with impaired glucose tolerance or Type 2 diabetes).
❏ Abnormal clotting factors (elevated fibrinogen and PAI-1).

Diabetes has other direct effects on the heart. Interstitial fibrosis, basement membrane thickening, and microaneurysm formation are recognized. Left ventricular contractility is reduced and this can lead to cardiac failure and arrythmias. This is known as diabetic cardiomyopathy. It is more common in those with microvascular disease. Arrythmias may be a cause of sudden death in young people with Type 1 diabetes. Ischaemic heart disease is more likely to be silent in those with diabetes. Angina and myocardial infarction may present with breathlessness, sweating, collapse, or malaise.

Improving cardiovascular risk

There should be an annual assessment of cardiovascular risk and this should include a record of blood pressure, blood glucose control, lipid profile, family history of arterial disease, adiposity, smoking habits, and albumin excretion. These risk factors should be managed aggressively. Where treatment changes are being made, follow-up will need to be more frequent. The patient should also be educated about the importance of each risk factor to be treated and the limitations and gains of therapy.

The National Institute of Clinical Excellence (NICE) has recommended that aspirin therapy should be offered to Type 2 diabetic patients who have more than a 15% risk of cardiac disease in the next 10 years and that it should be started after a target systolic blood pressure of 145 mmHg or lower has been achieved. *Table 12* presents the keys to reduction of cardiovascular risk in diabetic patients.

Lipid management

Ideally, fasting levels of total cholesterol, low-density [LDL]-cholesterol, HDL-cholesterol, and triglyceride should be measured annually. The target cholesterol level for Type 2 diabetes is currently recommended as <5.0 mmol/l (or an LDL-cholesterol of <3.0 mmol/l). If any of the damaging blood lipid parameters are elevated, it is essential to ensure that blood glucose is optimally controlled and that there is no other medical cause for the dyslipidaemia (e.g. hypothyroidism, liver or renal disease).

Lifestyle advice should be offered to help reduce blood lipids (diet, exercise, weight loss) and blood lipids should be repeated before commencing treatment.

Treatment with a statin drug is generally recommended for any diabetic patients with diabetes who have microalbuminuria, a strong family history of ischaemic heart disease, are from a high-risk ethnic group, have elevated blood pressure, have elevated blood lipids, or at least two features of the metabolic syndrome (raised blood pressure, high waist circumference, high triglycerides, low HDL-cholesterol). Treatment with a fibrate drug is indicated in cases of severe hypertriglyceridaemia.

Blood lipids should be regularly monitored after the initiation of therapy with the aim of achieving target levels of cholesterol and LDL-cholesterol. Some patients may require multiple therapies for control of abnormal blood lipids or cholesterol.

Blood pressure management

For patients with diabetes, blood pressure recordings should take place annually and at least six monthly for patients with established hypertension. Target blood pressure should be 140/80 mmHg. This may be reduced to 130/80 mmHg if there is another feature of the metabolic syndrome or evidence of micro-albuminuria or proteinuria.

If blood pressure is elevated, advice should be given on lifestyle changes that can reduce it such as a healthy diet, salt restriction, weight control, exercise, and glucose control. Raised blood pressure should be treated first with a low-dose thiazide or, where microalbuminuria or proteinuria is present, with an ACE inhibitor. Other medications that can be used include long-acting calcium channel blockers, angiotensin II receptor antagonists, beta-blockers and alpha-blockers. Multiple therapies are likely to be required, particularly in patients with features of the metabolic syndrome.

Obesity management

The management of overweight patients (body mass index [BMI] 25–30 kg/m^2) and obese patients (BMI >30 kg/m^2) with diabetes should include the recommendation of a low-energy diet with regular exercise. Dietary techniques include reducing the size of servings, adjusting the selection of food to encourage a healthy balanced diet, and avoidance of excessive unhealthy snacking. Dieting is not a physiological state and is difficult to adhere to for most. A moderate reduction in energy intake of 500–1000 kcal/day leads to a gradual loss of weight. Weight loss does become more difficult, however, as lean tissue is lost and energy expenditure reduces. Combination with an appropriate exercise regime is important at this stage. Very low calorie diets of less than 800 kcal/day are often in the form of a formula-based preparation. These should include appropriate vitamin and mineral supplements.

Low carbohydrate diets (e.g. the Atkins diet) have become fashionable since they combine the potential for satiety with rapid weight loss. There is no doubt that this can be an effective diet for weight loss although long-term health worries have not been fully explored. For diabetic patients on oral therapy or insulin it is essential that diets of this type are supervised, since the reduction in carbohydrate intake often requires a profound reduction in glucose-lowering therapy. For patients on insulin it may be necessary to reduce insulin dose by more than one-

---

Table 12 Keys to the reduction of cardiovascular risk in diabetes

❑ Optimization of blood glucose
❑ Control of blood pressure
❑ Control of blood lipids
❑ Reduction of thrombotic risk (antiplatelet therapy)
❑ Healthy diet
❑ Regular exercise
❑ Cessation of smoking
❑ Weight control, reduction of obesity

third on the day of commencing dietary modification. Patients with renal disease should not enter low carbohydrate dietary regimes since the proportionate increase in protein intake is likely to be damaging.

The antiobesity drugs orlistat, sibutramine, or rimonabant may have a role in the management of obesity in Type 2 diabetes. They should usually be reserved for patients who are established on appropriate diet and exercise regimes and have demonstrated the ability to lose some weight (2.5 kg over the preceding month).

Orlistat is a gastrointestinal lipase inhibitor that slows the rate of triglyceride digestion. This leads to an excessive amount of fat passing through to the faeces and side-effects of loose motion, diarrhoea, and even faecal incontinence are commonplace. These symptoms are exacerbated by a high dietary fat intake.

Weight loss should be assessed at 3 months and 6 months and discontinued if weight loss of less than 5% and 10% has occurred at these two time points. Therapy should usually be discontinued at 1 year.

Vitamin supplementation, particularly vitamin D, should be considered if there is a worry about loss of fat-soluble vitamins. Average additional weight loss is 2–4 kg.

Sibutramine is a centrally-acting serotonin and noradrenaline re-uptake inhibitor. It enhances the satiety response. It can lead to a small rise in blood pressure and pulse rate and should not be used in hypertensive patients. It is advised that patients taking sibutramine should have pulse rate and blood pressure monitored twice weekly for the first 3 months then monthly for 3 months and three monthly after that. Treatment should not exceed 1 year. Rimonabant is a newer centrally-acting appetite suppressant that works on the endo-cannabinoid system and has been shown to improve glycaemic control and stimulate weight loss. Oral therapy for obesity should be provided alongside arrangements for dietary counselling and behavioural/physical activity strategies to promote weight loss. It is not an answer to obesity if used in isolation.

DIABETES IN CHILDHOOD

Diabetes occurring in childhood is usually Type 1. However, in recent years there has been a worrying trend for Type 2 diabetes to present in teenage years. Hereditary forms of diabetes (maturity-onset diabetes of the young [MODY]), cystic fibrosis, Down's syndrome, and a few rare genetic syndromes listed below make up less than 5% of childhood diabetes:

❏ DIDMOAD syndrome (diabetes insipidus, diabetes mellitus, optic atrophy, deafness).
❏ Leprechaunism (growth retardation, dysmorphic facies, insulin resistance, reduced body fat, acanthosis nigricans).
❏ Rabson–Mendenhall syndrome (dysmorphic facies, insulin resistance, acanthosis nigricans).
❏ Congenital and acquired lipodystrophies (absence of fat, hepatomegaly, insulin resistance, hypertriglyceridaemia).

The incidence of Type 1 diabetes in childhood is increasing. There is currently an annual increase of around 3% in European countries. This increase is most marked in young children (<5 years). Those who develop diabetes in childhood can expect a reduction in life expectancy of around 20 years, with the possibility of complications before then.

Type 1 diabetes in childhood typically presents with polyuria, polydypsia, and weight loss. Fatigue, altered behaviour, infections (skin and urinary tract), generalized illness, and abdominal pain can also be presenting features.

A significant proportion of children with newly diagnosed diabetes will present as an emergency with DKA. The principles of management are the same as those in adults: resuscitation and airway management, replacement of fluid, insulin, and electrolytes with regular monitoring of conscious state, circulation, glucose concentration, acid-base state, and electrolytes. Fluid replacement and the rate of insulin infusion are dependent upon the age and size of the child. Younger children will require higher rates of insulin infusion for their body weight than older children.

Children with suspected Type 1 diabetes should be offered a same-day referral to a multidisciplinary diabetes team that can offer immediate diagnosis and care. Initial management can be from home or from within the hospital setting according to their age and needs. Children and their families should be offered a comprehensive educational package and 24 hour access to specialist advice. Emotional support may be required for both family and child.

Initially insulin requirements are low (the honeymoon period). Subsequently requirements increase, typically up to 1 unit/kg during the pubertal growth spurt. The most commonly used insulin regime in childhood is twice daily administration of a mixed preparation via an insulin pen. However, the introduction of new quick-acting insulin analogues has increased the use of basal bolus systems of insulin administration.

This is because the new analogues can be given immediately after a meal, reducing the risk of hypoglycaemia for an infant who then refuses to eat.

Insulin pump therapy has been introduced in an increasing number of children with erratic control and severe, recurrent hypoglycaemia.

An HbA1c level of less than 7.5% should be targeted in children with diabetes. This should be tested every 3–6 months. Children and their carers should be encouraged to monitor blood glucose. They should be educated to understand the effects of insulin, diet, and exercise and to adjust treatment to optimize glucose control. Preprandial glucose levels of 4–8 mmol/l and postprandial levels <10 mmol/l should be targeted.

Hypoglycaemia is extremely prevalent in children, particularly overnight, and should be avoided wherever possible. It is also a significant worry for parents of children with diabetes. Children and their carers should be educated about the management of hypoglycaemia and should have access to carbohydrate and blood glucose monitoring equipment. Children should be encouraged to wear a bracelet or carry identification indicating that they have diabetes. Hypoglycaemia is common but may be difficult to recognize, particularly in younger children who cannot communicate their symptoms so clearly. There is also evidence that children are less able to detect hypoglycaemia than adults. Consequently, severe hypoglycaemia is more common in children, with an incidence of about 0.2 episodes per patient-year. This rises to 0.6 episodes per patient-year in children under the age of 4 years.

Children may report classical autonomic and neuroglycopenic symptoms or may complain of headache, nausea, or nightmares. Alternatively, parents may recognize subtle features in their children that can be easily missed. These include:

❑ Irritability.
❑ Anger.
❑ Aggression.
❑ Attention deficit.
❑ Confusion.
❑ Bad behaviour.
❑ Impaired sleep.
❑ Drowsiness.
❑ Sweating.
❑ Pallor.

Severe hypoglycaemia may present with unconsciousness or seizures. Seizures are more prevalent in children than in adults. There is evidence that young children (<5 years) with recurrent severe episodes of hypoglycaemia are at increased risk of long-term neuropsychological changes. These include intellectual and cognitive development.

Children and their families should be encouraged to eat a healthy balanced diet and be able to understand the effects of different foods on blood glucose. They should be encouraged to consider a bedtime snack. Discussion about the timing and content of snacks should take place with a diabetes specialist. All children should be encouraged to exercise regularly and should be offered advice about restricted sports (e.g. scuba diving). They should be given information about precautions around exercise and adjusting food and insulin (outlined in Section 3). Children with diabetes have special needs. Together with their families, attention has to be paid to physical, psychological, intellectual, educational, and social development. All young people above the age of 6 months should be offered immunization with pneumococcal vaccine.

DIABETES IN ADOLESCENCE

The transition from childhood to adulthood poses particular difficulties for those with diabetes. There are physical, psychological, social, and educational problems that are more prevalent in this age group. Hormonal changes through puberty and the emotional effects relating to this time of life are reflected in a worsening of glycaemic control in the early to mid-teenage years. Emergency admissions and death rates are increased in this group. Young people with diabetes need support through the transition from childhood through adolescence to adulthood.

Young people should be informed about the specific effects of alcohol consumption. They should be encouraged not to smoke or offered help to stop. They should be advised of the risks and effects of substance abuse. The culture change that occurs on transition from paediatric to adult clinic can be dramatic and patients can feel unsupported. All young people with diabetes should experience a smooth transition from the paediatric diabetes service to the adult diabetes service via a young people's clinic. A range of psychological and social problems is more common in this age group. Emotional and behavioural difficulties, family conflict, eating disorders, and nonadherence to therapy are particularly commonplace. There needs to be timely and continuous access to mental health professionals in appropriate settings. Structured behaviour intervention support strategies for reducing family conflict are also necessary.

TYPE 2 DIABETES IN CHILDHOOD

Given that the complications of diabetes relate to the duration of the condition, the recent appearance of Type 2 diabetes in pubertal and postpubertal children is a worrying development. This condition was initially recognized in children from high-risk ethnic groups but is now seen in severely obese Caucasian children on both sides of the Atlantic. This increased incidence is directly related to the rise in childhood obesity. These children frequently have a family history of diabetes and may belong to a high-risk ethnic group (Asian, Afro-Caribbean or Middle-eastern descent). They are obese with features of insulin resistance such as polycystic ovarian syndrome or acanthosis nigricans. They are best managed in a similar manner to adults with Type 2 diabetes. The emphasis should be on lifestyle changes, tackling obesity, and addressing cardiovascular risk factors. Those who fail to achieve glycaemic goals with diet should initially be treated with metformin therapy.

MATURITY-ONSET DIABETES OF THE YOUNG (MODY)

MODY is a collection of syndromes that are characterized by an onset in childhood or early adulthood and account for about 1% of diabetes cases in Europe. Many cases go unrecognized. This genetically inherited group of conditions all occur as a result of a single gene defect, (six different types have currently been identified). Patients with this condition typically do not require require insulin or only require it in small doses, although β-cell dysfunction is typical and insulin resistance is not usually a feature.

Insulin treatment is not required and there is usually autosomal dominant transmission through at least two generations of family. The most common forms are mutations in transcription factors (75%) or the glucokinase enzyme (15%). The transcription factor mutations, of which the most common type is HNF1α, cause a progressive loss of β-cells. Sufferers develop the condition aged 10–30 years and can develop marked postprandial hyperglycaemia. Some require sulphonylurea tablets and others insulin therapy but there is little response to insulin-sensitizing drugs.

Glucokinase MODY typically leads to mild, stable fasting hyperglycaemia and is present from birth. It does not require medical intervention and is rarely associated with the typical microvascular complications of diabetes. Females should be advised to seek early assessment and monitoring during pregnancy.

PREGNANCY AND DIABETES

Although fetal and maternal mortality rates in diabetic pregnancy have fallen dramatically in the past 50 years, they still do not approximate outcomes in nondiabetic pregnancy. The key to improving outcome is optimal blood glucose control. Diabetes care should take place in a combined obstetric and diabetes clinic within a specialist setting. This care involves frequent review (2–4 weekly) throughout the course of the pregnancy.

There are a number of significant risks to mother and baby associated with diabetic pregnancy (*Tables 13, 14*). The teratogenic effects of diabetes relate strongly to the severity of hyperglycaemia during the important first 8 weeks of development.

Table 13 Increased risks associated with maternal diabetes in pregnancy

- ❏ Pre-eclampsia (twofold) and hypertension
- ❏ Polyhydramnios and preterm labour
- ❏ Worsening retinopathy/blindness
- ❏ Worsening nephropathy and proteinuria
- ❏ Caesarean section (nearly 50%)
- ❏ Unmasking coronary heart disease
- ❏ Urinary tract infections
- ❏ Heartburn and carpal tunnel syndrome

Table 14 Increased risks of maternal diabetes to the fetus

- ❏ Increased fetal growth (macrosomia)
- ❏ Congenital malformations (spina bifida, anencephaly, other CNS and cardiac malformations)
- ❏ Still birth (fourfold increase)
- ❏ Perinatal death
- ❏ Neonatal hypoglycaemia
- ❏ Neonatal respiratory distress syndrome (sixfold increase)
- ❏ Birth trauma
- ❏ Diabetes (2–6% risk with Type 1 diabetes)
- ❏ Neonatal jaundice
- ❏ Neonatal hypocalcaemia

GESTATIONAL DIABETES

Gestational diabetes is the development of diabetes or impaired glucose tolerance that is first diagnosed in a woman during pregnancy. In most women where the glucose intolerance or diabetes is actually precipitated by the pregnancy, glucose tolerance should return to normal in the postpartum period. The incidence of gestational diabetes in the UK is around 2%, but this rate is significantly increased in high-risk groups.

Gestational diabetes is becoming increasingly common because of increasing maternal age and obesity. It usually presents in the second or third trimester of pregnancy when insulin resistance is most high. The OGTT is used to diagnose gestational diabetes since fasting plasma glucose tends to decline during the early stages of pregnancy. A plasma glucose is checked 1 hour after administration of glucose. Screening for gestational diabetes with OGTT is carried out at 24–28 weeks and should be considered in those from the following high risk groups:

❏ Older women.
❏ Overweight or obese.
❏ Where there is recurrent glycosuria during pregnancy.
❏ Family history of diabetes in a first degree relative.
❏ High-risk ethnic group.
❏ Previous macrosomic infant (>4.5 kg), still-birth, or neonatal death.
❏ Glycosuria in a previous pregnancy.
❏ Polyhydramnios.
❏ Previous glucose intolerance.

The 75 g oral glucose tolerance test is used for screening. Screening should be done at the booking appointment where BMI is above 30, there is previous gestational diabetes, a first degree relative with diabetes, the ethnic background has a high prevalence of diabetes, or a previous baby has weighed >4.5 kg. For other risk factors an oral glucose tolerance test is carried out at 24–28 weeks. Gestational diabetes can be diagnosed if one or more of the following serum glucose values are met or exceeded:

❏ Fasting plasma glucose >7 mmol/l.
❏ Two hour post OGTT plasma glucose >7.8 mmol/l.

Oral drug therapy has generally been avoided in Type 2 diabetes although there is no evidence as yet that metformin or sulphonylureas are teratogenic.

Metformin is now being used during the later stages of pregnancy in some centres and many women fall pregnant on metformin now that it is used for the treatment of subfertility in polycystic ovarian syndrome. Sulphonylureas have previously been shown to be associated with severe neonatal hypoglycaemia, but second generation sulphonylureas do not have the same tendency to cross the placenta and are probably safe. For the majority of women who fail to achieve normal glucose levels during pregnancy the treatment is insulin. The decision to start insulin is dependent upon preprandial and postprandial home blood glucose monitoring. There is controversy as to which of these two is more important in terms of reducing fetal risk. The aim should be preprandial glucose levels of <5–6 mmol/l and postprandial glucose levels of <7–9 mmol/l. The principles of insulin use in gestational diabetes are similar to those in Type 1 patients on insulin (see later).

Gestational diabetes increases the risk of macrosomia in babies. It also confers an increased risk of subsequent Type 2 diabetes in mothers. This risk is at least 30%. It is therefore important to address recommend lifestyle interventions to address obesity, lack of exercise, and increased cardiovascular risk.

PLANNING PREGNANCY FOR THOSE WITH DIABETES

All diabetic pregnancies should be planned. It is therefore important for early and effective contraceptive advice to be given to all fertile women and girls with diabetes. Physical barrier methods such as the diaphragm or sheath are suitable for women with diabetes provided that they are used correctly. Intrauterine contraceptive devices appear to be safe and effective but should be avoided where there is evidence of pelvic infection. The oral combined contraceptive pill is effective and relatively safe with modern, low-dose oestrogen preparations. There is evidence that the combined pill may increase the risk of vascular events in susceptible patients. It should not be used in some patient groups:

❏ Age >35 years.
❏ Marked obesity.
❏ Uncontrolled hypertension.
❏ Hypertriglyceridaemia.
❏ Retinopathy.
❏ Nephropathy.
❏ Strong positive family history of heart disease.
❏ Cardiovascular disease.

The progesterone-only pill has no significant side-effects and is efficacious if taken correctly. It may be the best choice for many women with diabetes. Surgical sterilization or vasectomy can be considered for couples who do not wish to have further children or where it is contraindicated.

All women with diabetes should be made aware of the importance of prepregnancy counselling. It is essential that women seek advice before they attempt pregnancy rather than waiting until pregnancy has occurred. There are a number of important issues that need to be considered before pregnancy. The woman who wishes to become pregnant has to be made aware of how to plan pregnancy, what will be required during pregnancy, and why these measures are required. Prepregnancy counselling should include:
❑ An assessment of maternal risk (complications and comorbid disease).
❑ Advice on the risks of pregnancy (fetal and maternal).
❑ The initiation of insulin and stopping of glucose lowering tablets (for some).
❑ Advice on the importance of optimizing glucose control before and during pregnancy.
❑ The introduction of appropriate insulin regimes, frequent blood glucose monitoring, and dietary change (where necessary).
❑ The need for frequent antenatal visits.
❑ The need for early diagnosis of pregnancy and early antenatal care.
❑ Advice on stopping smoking.
❑ Advice on avoiding alcohol.
❑ The commencement of high-dose folate supplementation (5 mg/day).
❑ The stopping of ACE inhibitors and other teratogenic drugs.
❑ Advice on preconception contraception requirements.

Conditions such as proliferative retinopathy, renal failure, and previous myocardial infarction pose an extremely high risk to the mother. It may occasionally be sensible to advise against pregnancy or recommend additional treatment before conception.

ENDOCRINOLOGY

DISORDERS AFFECTING THE THYROID GLAND

Thyroid disease is common but may be symptomatic or asymptomatic. An annual screening of thyroid function blood tests should be carried out in the following patient groups:
❑ Symptomatic individuals.
❑ Atrial fibrillation, unexplained tachycardia, and hyperlipidaemia.
❑ Those receiving amiodarone or lithium therapy.
❑ Type 1 or Type 2 diabetes.
❑ Previous history of thyroid disease.
❑ Previous organ specific autoimmune disease (e.g. Addison's disease).
❑ Down's syndrome and Turner's syndrome.
❑ Family history of thyroid disease in an immediate relative.

THYROTOXICOSIS

This condition occurs where there is excessive thyroid hormone delivered to body tissues. It is usually due to hyperthyroidism, i.e. a hyperfunctioning of the thyroid gland. It much more commonly affects women than in men, in a ratio of 8:1. This increased prevalence probably relates to the presence of oestrogen although the mechanisms are unclear. Thyrotoxicosis affects 1 in 50 women at any given time. *Table 15* presents the common causes of thyrotoxicosis.

Table 15 Common causes of thyrotoxicosis

❑ Autoimmune disease, predominantly Graves' disease
❑ Toxic solitary thyroid nodule
❑ Toxic multinodular goitre
❑ Subacute viral (de Quervain's) thyroiditis
❑ Postpartum thyroiditis
❑ Excessive exogenous thyroid administration
❑ Drug-induced thyroiditis (principally amiodarone)
❑ Trophoblastic tumours secreting beta-HCG or ovarian teratoma
❑ Pituitary TSH adenoma
❑ Thyroid resistance syndrome
❑ Thyroid cancer (rare)

Table 16 Symptoms of thyrotoxicosis

- ❏ Shakiness
- ❏ Heat intolerance
- ❏ Palpitations
- ❏ Excessive sweating
- ❏ Mood disturbance
- ❏ Irritability
- ❏ Insomnia
- ❏ Hyperactivity
- ❏ Tiredness
- ❏ Weakness
- ❏ Breathlessness
- ❏ Weight loss or weight gain
- ❏ Increased appetite
- ❏ Increased stool frequency
- ❏ Polyuria
- ❏ Thirst
- ❏ Oligomenorrhoea
- ❏ Pruritus

Thyrotoxicosis can present with a multitude of disabling symptoms or may be symptom free. In the elderly patient it can present as unexplained weight loss or a change of behaviour. The more common symptoms are listed in *Table 16*.

Physical signs of thyroid overactivity are usually present. They may be masked however by the concominant use of beta-blocker therapy. In the absence of this drug treatment the first three physical signs are almost universal (*Table 17*). Where there are structural abnormalities of the thyroid gland these may be palpated in the neck. Causes of a palpable goitre include:
- ❏ Thyroid nodule.
- ❏ Multinodular thyroid gland.
- ❏ Graves' disease.
- ❏ Rarely thyroid malignancy.

Graves' disease

This is the commonest cause of thyrotoxicosis in the UK. It is an organ-specific autoimmune disorder more common in those with the HLA-DR3 phenotype.

Circulating antibodies bind to thyroid stimulating hormone (TSH) receptors activating them and stimulating excessive thyroid hormone release There are symptoms and signs that relate specifically to the presence of Graves' disease (**29, 30a & b**) (*Table 18*).

Table 17 Physical signs of thyroid overactivity

- ❏ Fine tremor
- ❏ Warm, moist palms
- ❏ Tachycardia/atrial fibrillation
- ❏ Eyelid retraction/lid lag
- ❏ Restlessness
- ❏ Hyper-reflexia
- ❏ Thinning of hair
- ❏ Palmar erythema
- ❏ Onycholysis
- ❏ Proximal muscle weakness/wasting
- ❏ Cardiac failure
- ❏ Psychosis

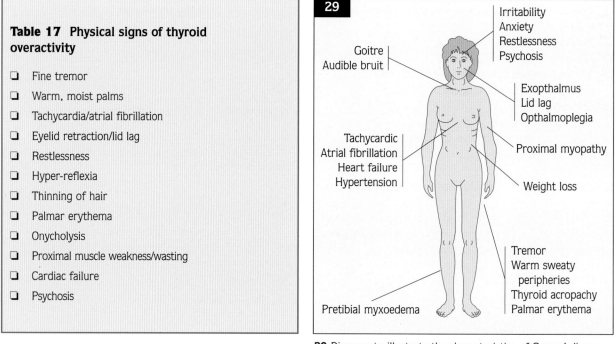

29 Diagram to illustrate the characteristics of Graves' disease.

Graves' ophthalmopathy

This is an ocular manifestation of Graves' disease. It is characterized by inflammation and lymphocytic infiltration of the extraocular muscles that can lead to fibrosis and tethering of the muscles. The condition is exacerbated by smoking and radioiodine therapy. There is an acute inflammatory phase during the early development of Graves' disease and a late phase that usually lags behind the clinical thyrotoxicosis. Clinical features of Graves' ophthalmopathy include:

❑ Dryness and grittiness.
❑ Eyelid retraction.
❑ Proptosis.
❑ Ophthalmoplegia.
❑ Optic neuropathy.

Significant proptosis should be investigated with an MRI scan of the orbit which typically shows enlargement of the extraocular muscles. Patients may complain of diplopia due to ophthalmoplegia and eye movement should be assessed. Patients with visual blurring or conjunctival pain should be referred for ophthalmology assessment in case of optic nerve damage, ophthalmoplegia, or corneal ulceration.

Pretibial myxoedema appears as raised, discoloured, and indurated skin typically on the shins. It is caused by the accumulation of glycosaminoglycans with a lymphoctic infiltrate. It can be disfiguring and occasionally painful.

Differential diagnoses

Sub-acute viral thyroiditis, also known as De Quervain's thyroiditis, typically presents with fever, neck pain, and a tender, enlarged thyroid gland. The patient may be thyrotoxic but may subsequently become hypothyroid. An erythrocyte sedimentation rate (ESR) is typically elevated and a radioisotope uptake scan shows reduced uptake of iodine by the thyroid gland. Postpartum thyroiditis typically occurs within 6 months of pregnancy and affects 5% of women. It may lead to subsequent hypothyroidism. An isolated autonomous thyroid nodule may be responsible for the excessive secretion of thyroid hormones (toxic thyroid nodule). These are typically benign. Another typically benign condition is the toxic multinodular goitre, characterized by thyrotoxicosis arising in a generalized nodular thyroid gland.

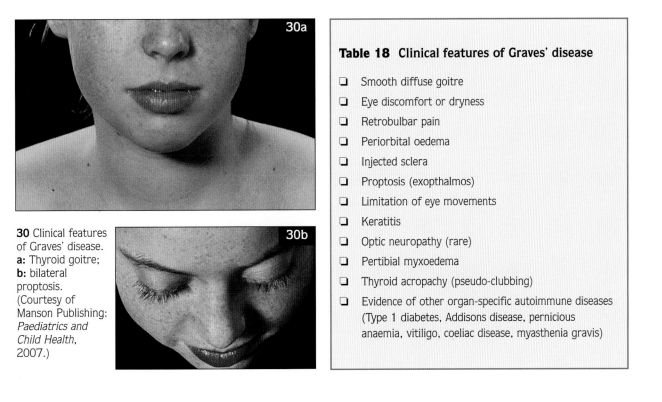

30 Clinical features of Graves' disease. **a:** Thyroid goitre; **b:** bilateral proptosis. (Courtesy of Manson Publishing: *Paediatrics and Child Health*, 2007.)

Table 18 Clinical features of Graves' disease

❑ Smooth diffuse goitre
❑ Eye discomfort or dryness
❑ Retrobulbar pain
❑ Periorbital oedema
❑ Injected sclera
❑ Proptosis (exopthalmos)
❑ Limitation of eye movements
❑ Keratitis
❑ Optic neuropathy (rare)
❑ Pertibial myxoedema
❑ Thyroid acropachy (pseudo-clubbing)
❑ Evidence of other organ-specific autoimmune diseases (Type 1 diabetes, Addisons disease, pernicious anaemia, vitiligo, coeliac disease, myasthenia gravis)

Investigation of thyrotoxicosis

1. Thyroid function tests should be performed. These should consist of a TSH assay combined with a free thyroxine (T4) and/or a free tri-iodothyronine (T3) assay. Typically there should be an elevation of T3 and T4 with suppression of TSH. In T3 thyrotoxicosis the T4 may be normal. In the rare case of a TSH-secreting adenoma, the free T4 and free T3 will be elevated but TSH levels will be normal or increased.

2. Thyroid antibodies are frequently found in autoimmune thyroid disease and should be checked. The three antibody types frequently tested are:
   ❑ Antithyroid peroxidase.
   ❑ Antithyroglobulin.
   ❑ TSH receptor antibodies.

Antibodies can be seen with variable specificity in Graves' disease or autoimmune hypothyroidism. Antithyroid peroxidase is present in the majority (>75%) of patients with Graves' or Hashimoto's disease, but TSH receptor antibodies are specific to Graves' disease.

3. Radioisotope scanning with ^{123}Iodine or ^{99}Technitium may be carried out to determine the cause of the thyrotoxicosis. *Table 19* presents the typical appearance of various conditions on a radioisotope scan. Thyrotoxicosis may also be associated with a normocytic anaemia, elevated alkaline phosphatase, and mild hypercalcaemia.

Secondary thyroid disease – TSH-secreting pituitary adenoma

This is a rare cause of hyperthyroidism and accounts for <1% of all functioning pituitary tumours. This diagnosis should be considered in all hyperthyroid patients, especially those with a diffuse goitre and no extrathyroidal manifestations of Graves' disease. The mean age at presentation is 41 years and it affects men and women equally. Most patients have the typical symptoms and signs of hyperthyroidism. Features include:
❑ A diffuse goitre in 95%.
❑ Visual field defects in 40%.
❑ Menstrual irregularity in 30%.
❑ Galactorrhoea in 30%.

The adenomas secrete TSH autonomously. TSH concentrations range from normal to markedly elevated (>500 mU/l). However, 'normal' values are inappropriately high in the presence of high serum T4 and T3 concentrations. In addition, serum TSH concentrations do not increase in response to thyroid releasing hormone (TRH) in the majority of patients. MRI examination of the pituitary should be performed in any hyperthyroid patient with a normal or high serum TSH concentration.

Patients with TSH-secreting adenomas and hyperthyroidism must be distinguished from those with the syndrome of resistance to thyroid hormone (RTH) (Refetoff's syndrome). Patients present with clinical hypothyroidism but with elevated thyroid hormone levels and normal or elevated TSH. Patients with RTH have variable tissue hypo-responsiveness to thyroid hormone due to a defect in the thyroid hormone receptor beta-gene. The following findings help to distinguish TSH-secreting adenomas from RTH:
❑ The serum sex hormone-binding globulin concentration (SHBG) is high in patients with TSH-secreting pituitary adenomas. The serum alpha-subunit concentration is normal in RTH but, as noted above, is often high in patients with TSH-secreting adenomas.
❑ The serum TSH concentration increases in response to TRH in patients with RTH, but not in most patients with TSH-secreting adenomas.
❑ Patients with RTH are more likely to have a fall in serum TSH concentrations in response to T3 (90% *vs.* 12–25%).

Table 19 Typical appearance of thyroid conditions on radioisotope scan

Diagnosis	Appearance
Graves' disease	Diffusely enlarged gland with increased uptake
Acute viral thyroiditis	Reduced uptake
Toxic thyroid nodule	A solitary area of increased uptake
Thyroid malignancy	Reduced uptake

HYPOTHYROIDISM

Hypothyroidism is a condition characterized by a deficiency of circulating thyroid hormones. There are a number of causes, as presented in *Table 20*. The commonest cause of chronic hypothyroidism is Hashimoto's disease. Antibodies and a T-cell response that result in inflammation and fibrosis of thyroid parenchyma cause this. Positive antibodies to thyroid peroxidase are usually found. This organ-specific autoimmune condition is commonly associated with other organ-specific autoimmune conditions, and patients should be screened for these.

Investigation of hypothyroidism

Primary hypothyroidism (thyroid underactivity caused by disease of the thyroid gland) is characterized by an elevation of serum TSH and a reduction in circulating free T4 or T3 levels. Secondary hypothyroidism is due to hypothalamic or pituitary disease and is characterized by a reduction in circulating T3 or T4 levels but no elevation of serum TSH. Subclinical hypothyroidism is a term used to denote raised TSH levels in the presence of normal circulating free T4 and free T4. These patients may progress to overt hypothyroidism (typically at a rate of 5% per year). Treatment should be initiated in those patients with a history of thyroid disease, positive thyroid antibodies, or with significantly elevated TSH (>10 mU/l). The remainder should be monitored with thyroid function tests (TFTs) every 3–6 months. A trial of thyroxine therapy can be considered in symptomatic patients or where the TSH is rising.

THYROID LUMPS (GOITRE, NODULES, AND MALIGNANCY)

Any localized or generalized enlargement of the thyroid gland requires a baseline TFT to assess thyroid gland activity. Any diffuse generalized enlargement of the gland is suggestive of autoimmune disease and requires antibody testing. Nodular or localized swelling of the gland requires imaging.

Iodine deficiency is the commonest cause of goitre worldwide. Clinically evident thyroid nodules (**31**) are present in about 10% of the UK population and may be single or multiple, as part of a multinodular goitre. Less than 5% are malignant but this becomes more common with increasing age. Autoimmune disease (Graves', Hashimoto's) also causes goitre.

Thyroid nodules are usually due to focal hyperplasia of thyroid follicular cells.

Table 20 Causes of hypothyroidism

Common causes
- ❑ Chronic autoimmune hypothyroidism (*Hashimoto's disease*)
- ❑ Postradioiodine therapy
- ❑ Postthyroid surgery
- ❑ Panhypopituitarism
- ❑ Transient hypothyroidism following subacute thyroiditis

Less common causes
- ❑ Congenital hypothyroidism, thyroid agenesis, thyroid hormone dysgenesis, Pendred's syndrome
- ❑ Atrophic thyroiditis
- ❑ Neoplastic infiltration
- ❑ Sarcoidosis
- ❑ Isolated TSH deficiency
- ❑ Drug-induced (amiodarone, lithium, iodides, phenylbutazone)
- ❑ Iodine deficiency
- ❑ Postradiation

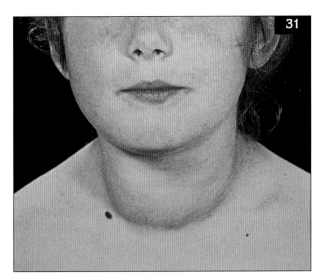

31 A discrete painless thyroid nodule in a young girl. (Courtesy of Manson Publishing: *Paediatrics and Child Health*, 2007.)

Clinical findings that increase the likelihood of thyroid malignancy include:
❏ Recent thyroid gland enlargement.
❏ A hard, nontender lump.
❏ Fixation to adjacent tissues.
❏ Associated lymphadenopathy.
❏ A hoarse voice.

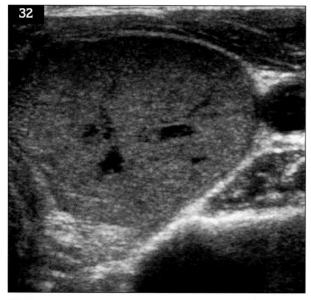

32 Ultrasound of thyroid gland showing a 4.7 × 2.2 × 2.2 cm thyroid nodule. (Courtesy of Dr J. Thomas, St Bartholomew's Hospital, London.)

Investigation of thyroid lumps

1. Ultrasound (**32**) scanning provides an indication of size and helps to differentiate between causes of an enlarged thyroid gland. *Table 21* presents the typical ultrasound findings in thyroid disease.
2. Fine-needle aspiration (FNA) cytology of thyroid nodules should be carried out on single nonactive nodules. This procedure should be repeated at 3–6 months since 5% of samples may be falsely negative. If FNA cytology is positive, the thyroid nodule should be surgically removed since there is a high risk of malignancy.
3. Computing tomography (CT) scanning should be carried out if there are symptoms suggestive of tracheal compression (**33**) or if thyroid malignancy is diagnosed. CT will evaluate retrosternal extension of the thyroid gland and any infiltration of local structures (vessels, trachea, oesophagus, and lymph nodes).

Thyroid malignancy

Cancer of the thyroid gland is uncommon, accounting for less than 1% of all malignancies. It affects women more often than men and is most frequently seen in the 5th decade of life. External irradiation is associated with an increased risk.

There are five malignancies that can arise in the thyroid gland. In order of frequency these are:
❏ Papillary carcinoma (70%).
❏ Follicular carcinoma (15%).
❏ Anaplastic carcinoma (5%).

Table 21 Typical ultrasound findings in thyroid disease

Ultrasound finding	Likely diagnosis
Diffusely enlarged gland	Graves' disease
Multiple nodules	Multinodular goitre
Single solid nodule	Benign or malignant thyroid nodule
Single cyst	Thyroid cyst or cystic nodule
Microcalcified nodule	Likely thyroid malignancy
Calcified thyroid gland	Possible medullary carcinoma of thyroid

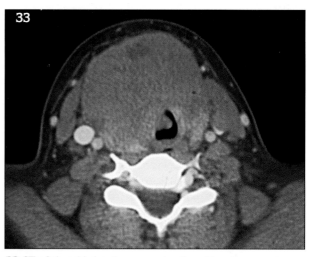

33 CT of thyroid showing a massive thyroid malignancy compressing and invading the trachea. (Courtesy of Dr J. Thomas, St Bartholomew's Hospital, London.)

❏ Medullary carcinoma (5%).
❏ Lymphoma (5%).

The prognosis for papillary and follicular carcinoma is good. Papillary carcinoma is confined to the thyroid in over 80% of cases. Local invasion occurs in the remainder with 1–2%, metastasizing via lymphatics to lymph nodes and lung. Follicular carcinoma is a tumour of thyroid epithelium. Metastases occurs in 15% of patients. It typically metastasizes to lung and bones. Anaplastic carcinoma is commonest in the 7th decade of life. Its growth is rapid and infiltrates local tissue aggressively. The long-term prognosis is poor with a 5-year survival rate of 5–10%. Medullary cell carcinoma is a tumour of parafollicullar C-cells secreting calcitonin and is frequently associated with Type 2 MEN (multiple endocrine neoplasia) syndrome. Diarrhoea is common as the presenting symptom. Circulating calcitonin levels are typically elevated. Lymphoma may be limited to the thyroid gland or be part of a systemic lymphoma. It presents with rapid enlargement of the thyroid gland. It is more common in women, age >40 years and in previous Hashimoto's disease.

PARATHYROID DISEASE
HYPERCALCAEMIA AND HYPERPARATHYROIDISM
Hypercalcaemia
Hypercalcaemia is a common clinical problem. Population studies have suggested a prevalence of about 3% in those over the age of 60 years. The clinical presentation may be asymptomatic or present with typical symptoms. Primary hyperparathyroidism and malignancy (especially solid tumours) account for 90% of all cases of hypercalcaemia. Other causes include:
❏ Sarcoidosis and other granulomatous diseases.
❏ Vitamin D intoxication.
❏ Familial hypocalciuric hypercalcaemia (FHH).
❏ Thiazide diuretics.
❏ Immobility.
❏ Renal failure.
❏ Addison's disease.

Hypercalcaemia affects a wide range of organ systems. The symptoms can be vague and nonspecific (*Table 22*); this has led to the phrase 'stones, bones, moans, and psychic groans' as a way of remembering the features of hypercalcaemia.

Symptoms associated with hypercalcaemia correlate to the concentration of calcium and the

Table 22 Symptoms of hypercalcaemia

❏ Polyuria
❏ Polydipsia
❏ Abdominal pain
❏ Reduced appetite
❏ Nausea and vomiting
❏ Constipation
❏ Lethargy
❏ Confusion
❏ Poor concentration
❏ Depressive illness

rapidity of onset of the hypercalcaemia. Since calcium is bound to albumin, the ionized calcium level can vary depending upon the albumin level (i.e. low albumin levels lead to higher ionized calcium). Therefore, the total calcium level needs to be corrected for albumin using the following formula:

$$\text{Corrected Ca}^{++} = \text{Ca}^{++} + 0.02 \times (40 - \text{serum albumin})$$

Investigations for hypercalcaemia
A detailed clinical history should be taken and a clinical examination (including breast examination) performed. Initial investigations should include:
❏ Chest X-ray.
❏ Serum calcium, phosphate.
❏ Urea and electrolytes.
❏ Liver biochemistry.
❏ Serum electrophoresis.

Further investigations may include the following:
1. In cases where malignancy is not likely, a serum parathyroid hormone (PTH) assay will need to be measured. This will give a diagnostic accuracy of 95%. The PTH will be inappropriately elevated (or occasionally in the upper normal range) in patients with primary or tertiary hyperparathyroidism. A low serum phosphate is also suggestive of hyperparathyroidism. The calcium concentration is frequently only mildly or moderately elevated in hyperparathyroidism, typically up to 3.5 mmol/l.

2. A 24-hour urinary calcium level should also be measured. If this is high and PTH levels are elevated, this confirms primary or tertiary hyperparathyroidism. However, if the urinary calcium is low, then the diagnosis may be FHH.

If the PTH is low, then the causative pathology is most likely to be a malignant process. The clinical features of the underlying cancer may be obvious (usually lung, breast, myeloma, lymphoma, or thyroid malignancy). Often the alkaline phosphatase is elevated.

Sarcoidosis and other granulomatous conditions produce PTH-like peptide that is dependent upon vitamin D supply. Vitamin D intoxication leads to elevation of 1,25-dihydroxycholecalciferol with suppressed PTH levels.

Other causes of hypercalcaemia
Malignancy
There are many tumours that can give rise to hypercalcaemia. The commonest are tumours of lung and breast as well as myeloma. Less frequently it can be seen with lymphoma and gastrointestinal, head, neck, and renal tumours.

The hypercalcaemia of malignancy is principally through two mechanisms that are not mutually exclusive:
1. Humeral hypercalcaemia – tumour cells produce parathyroid hormone related protein (PTHrP), which simulates the action of PTH. The presence of PTHrP can be checked for but only at a small number of specialist laboratories. Other growth factors such as transforming growth factor-α (TGF-α) and epidermoid growth factors are also potent activators of osteoclastic activity.
2. Direct osteolytic bone resorption – metastatic tumour cells, in common with osteoclasts, can cause direct resorption of bone. Consequently bone lysis can ensue. This is the main mechanism of action whereby myeloma and mestastatic bone disease cause hypercalcaemia. In osteolytic hypercalcaemia, the alkaline phosphatase level is usually markedly elevated. PTHrP may be elevated in malignancy.

Medication
Thiazide diuretics are known to cause hyper-calcaemia, by increasing the renal reabsorption of calcium. This is normally asymptomatic and is promptly corrected by stopping the medication.

Lithium may also cause hypercalcaemia through increased secretion of PTH.

Multiple endocrine neoplasia (MEN)
Multiple parathyroid tumours may coexist with tumours of the adrenal and thyroid glands. This is part of the MEN Type 2 syndrome. Parathyroid hyperplasia commonly occurs in MEN Type 1 syndrome in association with pancreatic, adrenal, and pituitary tumours.

Familial hypocalciuric hypercalcaemia (FHH)
This condition is inherited in an autosomal dominant fashion. The cause is a genetic defect of calcium sensing. Because the sensor is incorrectly set, the serum calcium is maintained at abnormally high levels. The family history, mild hypercalcaemia, detectable PTH level, and low urinary calcium excretion establish the diagnosis.

Hyperparathyroidism
The type of hyperparathyroidism can be divided into three:
❏ Primary: The abnormality lies with the parathyroid glands. The raised PTH level causes increased osteoclastic activity, with subsequent bone resorption.
❏ Secondary: PTH levels are raised due to any disease process which causes low calcium levels.
❏ Tertiary: This develops from secondary hyperparathyroidism where PTH secretion becomes autonomous, with excess PTH despite calcium levels returning to normal.

Primary hyperparathyroidism
There are three disorders causing primary hyper-parathyroidism:
1. A single benign parathyroid tumour (parathyroid adenoma) – 80% of cases.
2. Two or more enlarged glands (parathyroid hyperplasia) – 19% of cases.
3. Parathyroid cancer – 1% of cases.

If a diagnosis of primary hyperparathyroidism is made there should be investigations to localize the site of any parathyroid adenoma prior to surgery. These vary according to local practice but typically include 99mTc sestamibi scanning or thallium/ technetium subtraction scanning (**34a–c**). High-resolution ultrasound imaging, CT scanning or selective venous cannulation with concurrent measurement of PTH levels may be used where a parathyroid adenoma cannot be identified. None of these investigations has a sensitivity of more than 90% and often a combination of investigations is used.

If the site of the adenoma cannot be confirmed it may be necessary to carry out an MRI scan of neck and mediastinum to locate aberrant glands. Selective venous sampling of neck veins for parathyroid hormone can also localize the site of the lesion. Frequently exploratory neck surgery is required to localize the adenoma.

Secondary hyperparathyroidism
In this condition the parathyroid glands are secreting excess PTH in response to an initial low blood calcium level. The main causes of this are:

- ❏ Renal failure. There is failure to convert 25-cholecalciferol into 1,25-cholecalciferol, the active form of vitamin D. This means that the intestine absorbs calcium less readily from the diet resulting in a low serum calcium. The failing kidney also fails to excrete enough phosphate. Both of these factors contribute to an increase in secretion of PTH.
- ❏ Malabsorption. If there is a generalized malabsorption of nutrients from the diet, e.g. coeliac disease, the result is a low serum calcium and a subsequent increase in PTH release.
- ❏ Vitamin D and calcium deficiency. A diet deficient in calcium or vitamin D (required to absorb calcium) leads to low serum calcium and increased PTH release.

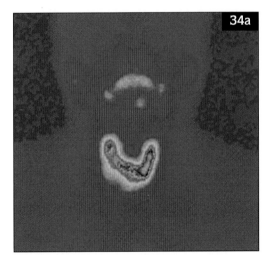

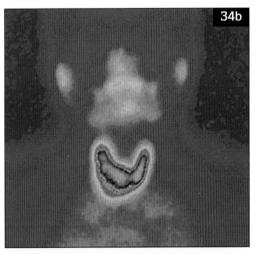

34 Parathyroid subtractions scans; (**a**) shows iodine uptake by a multi-nodular thyroid gland; (**b**) MIBI image taken up by the thyroid and parathyroids; (**c**) shows the subtraction image (MIBI minus iodine) revealing a right lower parathyroid adenoma. (Courtesy of Dr J. Thomas, Bartholomew's Hospital, London.)

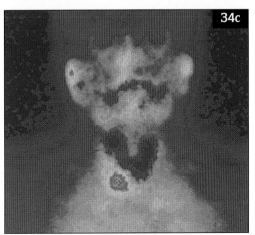

Tertiary hyperparathyroidism

Occasionally, if the causes of secondary hyper-parathyroidism persist for some time, one parathyroid gland may become autonomous. The cells start producing excessive amounts of PTH even if the stimulus of low calcium is removed (e.g. after medical treatment). This is tertiary hyperpara-thyroidism and is seen most commonly in patients with renal failure.

HYPOCALCAEMIA AND HYPOPARATHYROIDISM

The causes of hypocalcaemia are presented in *Table 23*. In hypoparathyroidism, the parathyroid glands do not secrete adequate PTH, for a variety of causes (*Table 24*). This results in a low blood calcium level (hypocalcaemia) where blood calcium is less than 2.25 mmol/l (10 mg/100 ml).

Hypocalcaemia causes a variety of symptoms that do not typically occur unless the calcium is less than 2.0 mmol/l:

- Tingling and numbness of feet, hands, and mouth (perioral parasthesia).
- Cramps.
- Muscle spasms.
- Seizures.
- Muscle weakness.

Clinical findings include signs of neuromuscular irritability:

1. Chvostek's sign. Tapping of the facial nerve just in front of the ear induces a twitching of the corner of the mouth.
2. Trousseau's sign. Inflation of a sphygmomanometer on the upper arm to above systolic blood pressure for more than 3 minutes induces a spasm in forearm muscles (carpo-pedal spasm).

Essential blood investigations for hypocalcaemia include:

- Calcium
- Phosphate.
- PTH.
- Vitamin D.
- Magnesium.

The presence of a low or normal PTH concentration in the presence of hypocalcaemia suggests a failure of PTH secretion. If pseudohypoparathyroidism is suspected, then the modified Ellsworth–Howard test should be performed (see *Table 24*).

Table 23 Causes of hypocalcaemia

- Hypoparathyroidism
- Low albumin – any reason for a low serum albumin will cause low serum calcium due to the calcium particles not being carried properly in the blood, allowing them to be excreted and lost
- Alkalosis – increased albumin binding
- Acute pancreatitis
- Osteomalacia
- Vitamin D deficiency
- Renal failure
- Drugs – ketoconazole, calcitonin, phosphate

Table 24 Causes of hypoparathyroidism

- Surgical removal (typically after procedures for thyroid disease or neck malignancy)
- Autoimmune disease – seen as part of polyglandular autoimmune syndrome Type 1 (hypoparathyroidism, adrenal insufficiency, thyroid disease, and diabetes mellitus)
- Infiltration with malignancy
- Irradiation
- Failure of development – inherited deficiency or as part of Di George syndrome
- Hypomagnesaemia
- Pseudohypoparathyroidism. The parathyroid hormone is normal or increased. It is due to a genetic defect as a result of tissue insensitivity to PTH. Calcium levels, therefore, remain low. In this condition there is a failure of cyclic AMP response to an infusion of parathyroid hormone (the modified Ellsworth–Howard test)

OTHER BONE DISORDERS

Osteoporosis

Osteoporosis is a condition where there is reduction of skeletal bone. It is associated with a reduction in bone mineral density and structural integrity. It is associated with an increased risk of bone fracture, particularly of

the wrist, hips, and vertebrae. These fractures frequently occur despite low trauma. Osteoporosis is more common in women of postmenopausal age, cigarette smokers, those who consume alcohol, have poor intake of calcium, and who do not carry out weight-bearing exercise. Other causes include:
❏ Testicular or ovarian failure (including early menopause, Turner's syndrome, and Klinefelter's syndrome).
❏ Low oestrogen states (including prolactinoma and anorexia nervosa).
❏ Endocrine disease (including Cushing's disease, hyperparathyroidism, thyrotoxicosis, and hypopituitarism).
❏ Gastrointestinal disease (including coeliac disease, malabsorption, and inflammatory bowel disease).
❏ Liver and renal disease.
❏ Drug-induced (including long duration, high-dose corticosteroids, anticonvulsants, long-term heparin, cyclosporin).
❏ Inherited disorders (including osteogenesis imperfecta, Marfan's syndrome, homocystinuria).

Investigation for osteoporosis
Investigations are carried out in those who present with a typical fracture or who are at increased risk of osteoporosis. Major risk facors are untreated hypogonadism, long-term high-dose glucocorticoid use (typically more than 7.5 mg prednisolone for a duration longer than 6 months), other organ disease as above, or osteopenia on routine X-ray imaging.

Bone densitometry is the investigation of choice. Bone mineral density is measured at the hip and lumbar spine using dual X-ray absorptiometry (DEXA scanning). Measurements are more reliable at the hip since spinal degeneration may artificially elevate the apparent bone mineral density. The T score is the standardized unit for measuring bone mineral density. A T score of −1 to −2.5 equates to a bone mineral density of 1–2.5 standard deviations below the age-matched mean and corresponds to osteopenia. Osteoporosis is defined as a T score >−2.5. If osteoporosis is diagnosed it is important to exclude the major causes outlined above.

Osteogenesis imperfecta
This is an inherited form of osteoporosis in which there is defective collagen formation. It presents in childhood. Other physical findings include:
❏ Blue sclerae.

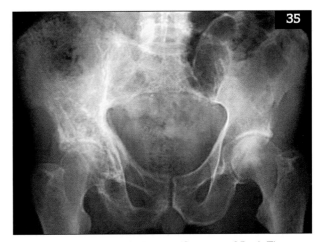

35 Pelvic X-ray of Paget's disease. (Courtesy of Dr J. Thomas, St Bartholomew's Hospital, London.)

❏ Dental abnormalities.
❏ Loss of hearing.

The condition may be recognized on X-ray through generalized osteopenia, multiple fractures, and deformity or abnormally-shaped long bones.

Paget's disease
Paget's disease is a condition that predominantly affects those aged >55 years. It affects 2% of the population and is more common in men. Typically there is hyperactivity of bone resorbing osteocleast cells and subsequent overactivity of osteoblasts. This leads to disorganized bone formation with a disturbed internal architecture. The bones most commonly affected are:
❏ Pelvis.
❏ Vertebrae.
❏ Skull.
❏ Femur.
❏ Tibia.

Affected bones are more prone to bend and fracture (this occurs in 70% of sufferers). Bone pain is the commonest feature. Secondary effects include arthritis and nerve compression including sensori-neural deafness. The diagnosis of Paget's disease is usually established radiologically on X-ray (**35**):
❏ Lytic lesions in skull and long bones.
❏ Cortical thickening.
❏ Lucency of bone.
❏ Increased bone size.
❏ Bony sclerosis.

Serum alkaline phosphatase is usually elevated and may correspond well to the activity of the disease. Radiosotope bone scanning can be used to help to assess the extent of the disease. Serious complications of Paget's disease include:
❏ Deafness.
❏ Spinal cord compression (rare).
❏ Osteosarcoma developing in affected bone.

Rickets and osteomalacia

Rickets (**36**) occurs in children where the skeleton is still growing. There is inadequate mineralization of new bone at the growth plates. Osteomalacia is inadequate mineralization of mature adult bone. The commonest cause is vitamin D deficiency; other causes are listed in *Table 25*. The clinical features of rickets/osteomalacia include:
❏ Bone pain.
❏ Deformity.
❏ Fracture.
❏ Proximal myopathy.
❏ Growth retardation (rickets).

Vitamin D deficiency leads to low levels of serum calcium and phosphate with an appropriate increase in PTH levels. Low levels of 25-hydroxy vitamin D and 1,25-dihydroxy vitamin D can be measured directly. Where the cause of osteomalacia is renal failure the results are similar except that phosphate is retained (and therefore elevated) and 25-hydroxy vitamin D levels are normal. (In order to be activated, vitamin D is first 25-hydroxylated in the liver and then 1-α-hydroxylated in the kidney). X-ray features of rickets include bowing of the long bones and widening of the epiphyseal growth plates.

DISORDERS AFFECTING THE ADRENAL GLANDS
ADRENAL HORMONE EXCESS
Cushing's syndrome
Cushing's syndrome is a condition characterized by excessive exposure to glucocorticoids. This may be cortisol hormone from the adrenal gland(s) or exogenous steroids. *Table 26* presents the causes of Cushing's syndrome.

The commonest cause of Cushing's syndrome is iatrogenic due to the long-term exogenous administration of oral corticosteroids, e.g. prednisolone. It is also possible to become 'cushingoid' with excessive doses of steroid administered via the inhaled, topical, or intranasal routes.

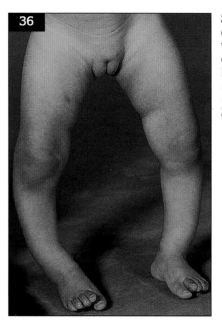

36 Rickets in a child (genu varum). (Courtesy of Manson Publishing: *Paediatrics and Child Health*, 2007.)

Table 25 Causes of rickets/osteomalacia and vitamin D deficiency

Causes of rickets/osteomalacia
❏ Vitamin D deficiency
❏ Renal failure
❏ Vitamin D-resistant rickets (inherited as X-linked hypophosphataemia)
❏ Malignancy (most commonly prostate cancer, CLL, myeloma)
❏ Inherited vitamin D receptor defects
❏ Fanconi syndrome
❏ Renal tubular acidosis

Causes of vitamin D deficiency
❏ Poor sunlight (most common in housebound, elderly, and Asian women)
❏ Poor diet (more common in vegetarians/vegans)
❏ Malabsorption states
❏ Phenytoin use (increased catabolism of vitamin D)
❏ Postgastric surgery

Cushing's syndrome that is not due to exogenous steroids is more common in women than men (3:1) and can present at any age (most commonly 3rd and 4th decades of life). It is rare, with an incidence of 0.2% of the population per

37 Diagram to illustrate the characteristics of Cushing's syndrome.

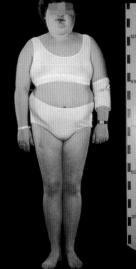

37

Depression
Psychosis

Proximal
muscle
wasting
Thin skin
Easy bruising
Hypertension

Moon face
Plethoric
Acne

Buffalo hump
Kyphosis
Fractures

Central obesity
Purple striae
Diabetes

Oedema
Skin infections

Table 26 Causes of Cushing's syndrome

❑ Iatrogenic Cushing's: exogenous administration of steroids (oral, inhaled, topical)
❑ Pseudocushings: excessive alcohol intake, severe depression
❑ ACTH-dependent Cushing's: pituitary adenoma (Cushing's disease), ectopic ACTH or CRH secretion
❑ ACTH-independent Cushing's: adrenal adenoma, carcinoma, or nodular hyperplasia

---

Table 27 Clinical features of Cushing's syndrome

❑ Rounded plethoric face
❑ Hirsutism
❑ Central obesity
❑ Proximal muscle weakness
❑ Acne
❑ Thinning of hair
❑ Thinning of skin/easy bruising
❑ Purple pigmented striae (abdomen, breasts, axillae, thighs) (**39**)
❑ 'Buffalo hump'
❑ Menorrhagia
❑ Mood disturbance
❑ Psychosis

38 Central obesity in Cushing's syndrome. (Courtesy of Manson Publishing: *Paediatrics and Child Health*, 2007.)

38

39 Abdominal striae in Cushing's syndrome. (Courtesy of Manson Publishing: *Paediatrics and Child Health*, 2007.)

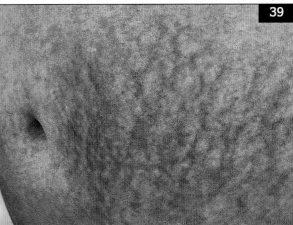

39

year. Cushing's syndrome is most frequently associated with an ACTH-secreting adenoma of the pituitary gland (pituitary-dependent Cushing's disease). It may also be due to a cortisol-secreting tumour of the adrenal gland or ACTH/cortico-trophin releasing hormone (CRH) secretion from an ectopic site. Untreated Cushing's disease has a 5-year mortality rate of 30% due to cardiovascular, metabolic, and infective complications.

The patient with Cushing's syndrome may have a typical 'lemon-on-sticks' appearance brought about by central obesity combined with loss of proximal musculature (**37**, **38**). Clinical features are listed in *Table 27*.

Examination and investigations of the cushingoid patient may reveal the following metabolic abnormalities:

- ❏ Hypertension (present in more than 60% of patients).
- ❏ Diabetes mellitus/impaired glucose tolerance (present in more than 30% of patients).
- ❏ Osteoporosis.
- ❏ Cardiovascular or other circulatory disease.

Specific investigations for Cushing's syndrome
Investigations for Cushing's syndrome should be considered in 3 stages:

1. Screening tests to exclude most 'normal' subjects.
2. Diagnostic tests to determine whether Cushing's syndrome is present.
3. Tests to determine the underlying cause.

Screening tests to exclude most 'normal' subjects
- ❏ 24-hour urinary free cortisol. This test should be repeated if normal since the false negative rate is 5%. There is a small number of patients with cyclical Cushing's in whom cortisol production is erratic. These patients may be missed without repeat testing or combining screening tests.
- ❏ Overnight dexamethasone suppression test. 1 mg of oral dexamethasone is ingested at midnight and a serum cortisol measurement taken at 9 am. There should be suppression of serum cortisol (<50 nmol/l). The false negative rate is 2%. False positive rates are high.
- ❏ Midnight cortisol. In Cushing's syndrome, there is a loss of circadian rhythm of cortisol secretion (7). In normal subjects the midnight level should be <50 nmol/l.

These tests may be positive in patients with pseudocushing's, where patients are obese, depressed, or consume excessive alcohol.

Diagnostic tests to determine whether Cushing's syndrome is present
- ❏ Low-dose dexamethasone suppression test. Dexamethasone (0.5 mg) is given orally 6 hourly for 48 hours. A 9 am cortisol at 48 hours should be suppressed (<50 nmol/l).
- ❏ Rarely, an insulin stress test to induce hypoglycaemia and stimulate cortisol secretion (see Pituitary disease, page 70).

Drugs that increase dexamethasone metabolism, e.g. phenytoin, can lead to false positives and should be avoided. Pseudocushing's can occasionally lead to false positives.

Tests to determine the underlying cause
- ❏ Serum ACTH level. Low levels (<20 ng/l) indicate a primary adrenal cause.

Very high levels (>200 ng/l) indicate an ectopic source of ACTH production (usually accompanied by hypokalaemia and rapid onset of symptoms). Intermediate/high levels indicate pituitary or ectopic ACTH production.

- ❏ High-dose dexamethasone suppression test. This is similar to the low-dose suppression test except that 2 g of dexamethasone is given 6 hourly. In pituitary-dependent Cushing's disease, the cortisol levels suppress to <50% that of basal levels. This does not occur with ectopic ACTH production. However, there is a 10% overlap of false negative and false positives.
- ❏ Pituitary MRI scan. MRI after gadolinium enhancement localizes ACTH-secreting microadenomas of the pituitary gland. The false positive rate is 10%.
- ❏ Pituitary hormone blood tests. Excessive cortisol can suppress the thyroid, gonadal, and GH axes.
- ❏ CT scan or MRI scan of adrenal glands. This is useful where an adrenal cause is suspected.
- ❏ Chest X-ray. This is important when ectopic ACTH production is suspected. Occasionally CT or MRI of neck, chest, and abdomen. Imaging is looking for sources of ectopic ACTH secretion.

Pituitary-dependent Cushing's disease
Approximately 70% of endogenous Cushing's syndrome (i.e. not due to exogenous use of steroids) is due to an ACTH-secreting adenoma of the pituitary gland (Cushing's disease). If Cushing's disease is suspected as a result of these investigations, bilateral inferior petrosal sinus sampling should be performed. This involves the measurement of ACTH centrally and peripherally. Sampling is combined with administration of CRH to stimulate ACTH production. A ratio of central to peripheral ACTH >3:1 indicates a pituitary cause and can help to localize the lesion to the left or right side.

Adrenal Cushing's syndrome

Adrenal tumours account for 20% of Cushing's syndrome. They are commonest in women and in the 4th and 5th decades of life. 60% are due to a benign adenoma. A small number (<2%) are secondary to nodular hyperplasia. The remainder are caused by adrenal carcinoma. Adrenal carcinoma usually has a more abrupt onset and may lead to masculinizing effects in women.

CT or MRI scanning of the adrenal glands gives good visualization. Carcinomas are usually larger tumours (typically >5 cm) and may exhibit calcification.

Ectopic ACTH syndrome

This is frequently due to malignancy but can be associated with phaeochromocytoma (see below). The commonest tumours associated with ectopic ACTH are:
- Small cell carcinoma of the lung.
- Lung, pancreatic, gut, or thymus carcinoid syndrome.
- Medullary carcinoma of the thyroid.

Ectopic ACTH syndrome is commonly associated with hypokalaemia and hypertension. Investigations should include chest X-ray, CT or MRI scan of the neck, chest, and abdomen, urinary 5-hydroxyindole acetic acid (5-HIAA) collections and serum calcitonin. Occasionally, selective venous sampling of thoracic veins can help determine the site of excess ACTH secretion.

Phaeochromocytoma

Phaeochromocytomas are rare tumours of the adrenal medulla that secrete catecholamines. 10% of catecholamine-secreting tumours can be seen elsewhere, most commonly in the paravertebral sympathetic nervous tissue. These are called paraganglioneuromas and are more likely to be malignant. These tumours occur equally in either sex and are most common in the 3rd and 4th decades of life. 10% are found in familial syndromes (typically Type 2 MEN syndrome); 10% are malignant and 10% are unilateral. Catecholamine secretion is usually adrenaline or noradrenaline and less commonly dopamine.

Although rare, young patients with unexplained hypertension, typical symptoms, or a family history of MEN should be screened for phaeochromocytoma.

Clinical features include:
- Persistent or paroxysmal hypertension, postural hypotension.
- Sweats.
- Flushes.
- Nervousness.
- Palpitations, chest pain, breathlessness.
- Fever.
- Headache.
- Abdominal pain, nausea.

Patients may present acutely with an adrenergic crisis precipitated by drugs, surgery, or exercise.

Investigating phaeochromocytoma

The screening test of choice is 24-hour urine collection for catecholamines. This should be repeated on at least one further occasion since this increases the sensitivity to nearly 100%. The reliability of the test increases if the urine is collected during an attack. Plasma catecholamines can be performed but are only useful to exclude the diagnosis during a symptomatic attack. A large number of drugs can interfere with catecholamine results and should ideally be stopped for several days prior to testing. These include:
- Tricyclic antidepressants.
- Phenothiazides.
- Metoclopramide.
- Levodopa.
- Monoamine oxidase inhibitors (MAOIs).
- ACE inhibitors.
- Beta-blockers.

Pentolinium or clonidine suppression tests are occasionally performed in patients with borderline catecholamine levels. MRI imaging of the adrenal glands and abdomen will demonstrate the majority (90%) of tumours. 123I-MIBG (meta-iodobenzyl-guanidine) scanning is positive in only 75% of phaeochromocytomas but may demonstrate extra-adrenal tumours not visualized on MRI scanning.

Mineralocorticoid excess – Conn's syndrome and related conditions

Excessive mineralocorticoid production can be due to either primary hyperaldosteronism where there is autonomous secretion of mineralocorticoid hormone or secondary hyperaldosteronism where there is increased secretion in response to ACTH or angiotensin II. Causes of excessive mineralocorticoid production are presented in *Table 28*.

Primary hyperaldosteronism is rare and is most commonly due to a unilateral adrenal adenoma (Conn's syndrome). It is more common in women and in the 3rd–6th decade. Adrenal carcinoma and bilateral adrenal hyperplasia can present with similar features.

Excessive aldosterone causes sodium retention with potassium and hydrogen ion loss at distal renal tubules. Patients with Conn's present with uncontrolled hypertension, frequently with a hypokalaemic alkalosis. This can lead to symptoms of polyuria, cramps, muscle weakness, parasthesia and, occasionally, tetany. Hypokalaemia is less common in patients with nodular hyperplasia of the adrenal glands.

Investigations for Conn's syndrome and related conditions should be carried out in young patients with hypertension, patients with unexplained resistant hypertension, and in patients with hypertension and unexplained hypokalaemia. Screening tests should include serum potassium, urinary potassium excretion, and a serum aldosterone:renin ratio. In patients with Conn's syndrome, the serum potassium is frequently low (70% of normal).

Urinary potassium excretion >30 mmol in 24 hours is consistent with the diagnosis. All other causes of hypokalaemia should be excluded before this diagnosis is excluded (e.g. vomiting, diarrhoea, diuretic use, laxative abuse). A ratio of aldosterone (pmol/l) to plasma renin activity (ng/ml/h) which is greater than 750 suggests primary hyperaldosteronism. It is important that serum potassium is normalized with supplements prior to this measurement. The test should be carried out in the morning in an upright position. Concominant antihypertensive medication should be stopped prior to the test.

The diagnostic investigation for Conn's disease is the measurement of plasma aldosterone, renin, and cortisol after lying horizontal overnight and after maintaining an upright posture for 4 hours. In normal individuals and in those with adrenal hyperplasia aldosterone levels and plasma renin activity (PRA) are increased on standing. In patients with an aldosterone-secreting adrenal adenoma, the aldosterone response is controlled more by ACTH secretion than posture so aldosterone levels fail to rise significantly. In addition, PRA is suppressed so does not increase in response to posture.

The ACE inhibitor test can help to differentiate between an adrenal nodule and hyperplasia. ACE inhibitors lead to a fall in aldosterone secretion 60 minutes after administration in hyperplasia but not where there is an adrenal adenoma. Serum cortisol is checked during the test to ensure that a circadian rhythm of cortisol secretion exists. If it does not this invalidates the test. Urinary 18-hydroxycortisol levels are also elevated in Conn's disease.

CT or MRI scanning of the adrenal glands identifies the majority of adenomas. In nodular hyperplasia, the glands may appear enlarged and nodular. Adrenal carcinoma (**40**) is more likely in tumours that are larger than 5 cm diameter or where there is local invasion seen on imaging.

Other available investigations include radio-labelled cholesterol uptake scanning (following administration of dexamethasone) and bilateral adrenal vein sampling for aldosterone levels to determine the side of the lesion.

Secondary hyperaldosteronism

Excessive mineralocorticoid secretion can be due to activation of the renin–angiotensin system or excessive ACTH. Causes include laxative or diuretic abuse, dehydration, renovascualr hypertension, and renin-secreting tumours. These conditions can be divided into those that cause hypertension and those that do not (*Table 29*).

11β-hydroxysteroid dehydrogenase deficiency

This is a rare condition that mimics hyperaldosteronism and is due to stimulation of distal nephron mineralocorticoid receptors by cortisol. It is usually seen in children. PRA and aldosterone are suppressed. Treatment is with dexamethasone to suppress ACTH secretion

ADRENAL HORMONE DEFICIENCY

Adrenal hormone deficiency may be due to primary adrenal disease (Addison's disease) or be secondary to a dysfunctional pituitary gland or hypothalamus.

Primary adrenal insufficiency – Addison's disease

Causes of Addison's disease are presented in *Table 30*. The commonest cause by far in the UK is autoimmune adrenalitis. Addison's disease is more common in women (2:1, female:male). Adrenal cortex antibodies are seen in the majority of patients.

Occasionally, this condition is seen as part of an autoimmune polyglandular syndrome. Type 1 auto-immune polyglandular syndrome is an autosomal recessive condition associated with a number of autoimmune conditions:

- ❑ Addison's disease.
- ❑ Hypoparathyroidism.
- ❑ Hypothyroidism.
- ❑ Ovarian/testicular failure.
- ❑ Chronic mucocutaneous candidiasis.
- ❑ Rarely, pernicious anaemia, chronic active hepatitis, and hypopituitarism.

Table 28 Causes of excessive mineralocorticoid production

- ❑ Aldosterone-secreting adrenal adenoma (Conn's syndrome)
- ❑ Aldosterone-secreting adrenal carcinoma
- ❑ Bilateral adrenal hyperplasia
- ❑ Secondary hyperaldosteronism
- ❑ Renal tubular disease
- ❑ Excessive liquorice ingestion
- ❑ Congenital adrenal hyperplasia

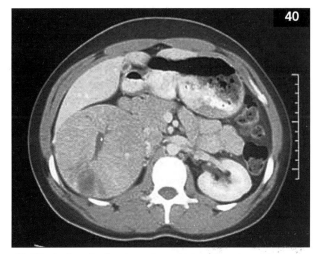

40 CT of adrenals showing a large (14 × 10 cm), heterogenous, right adrenal mass, consistant with malignancy (adrenocortical carcinoma). (Courtesy of of Dr J. Thomas, St Bartholomew's Hospital, London.)

Table 29 Causes of secondary mineralocorticoid excess

With hypertension
- ❑ Renovascular disease (most commonly atherosclerosis or fibromuscular hyperplasia)
- ❑ Renin-secreting tumours
- ❑ Accelerated hypertension
- ❑ Cushing's disease

Without hypertension
- ❑ Sodium-wasting syndromes (renal failure, renal tubular acidosis, volume depletion, diuretic use, laxative abuse)
- ❑ Liver cirrhosis
- ❑ Bartter's syndrome

Table 30 Causes of primary adrenal insufficiency

- ❑ Autoimmune – isolated or part of polyglandular condition
- ❑ Malignancy – lung, breast, renal metastases, and lymphoma
- ❑ Infiltration – sarcoid, amyloid, haemochromatosis
- ❑ Infection – tuberculosis, fungal, human immunodeficiency virus-related infections
- ❑ Vascular – infarction or haemorrhage
- ❑ Iatrogenic – ketoconazole, adrenalectomy
- ❑ Congenital adrenal hyperplasia – 21-hydroxylase deficiency
- ❑ Congenital – adrenoleukodystrophy

Inadequate ACTH results in atrophy of the zona fasciculata and deficient cortisol production. There are also reduced androgens in women. Unlike Addison's disease there is absence of pigmentation and a lack of mineralocorticoid deficiency. Hypokalaemia and postural symptoms are therefore not typically present.

Congenital adrenal hyperplasia (CAH)
Classical CAH
CAH represents a group of syndromes where there is absence or a reduced level of enzymes involved in steroid synthesis. There is a range of enzyme deficiencies that lead to different clinical diseases. In the most common form of CAH, which accounts for more than 90% of CAH, there is a deficiency of the 21-hydroxylase enzyme (**43**). As with the other forms of CAH, 21-hydroxylase deficiency is transmitted as an autosomal recessive disorder.

In this form of CAH, the production of cortisol and aldosterone is low while testosterone is produced normally. The lack of negative feedback from cortisol results in an increase in ACTH production, which drives the steroid production pathway resulting in an increase in testosterone production. Sufferers with signs only of androgen excess but no salt-wasting are said to have the simple virilizing form of 21-hydroxylase deficiency. In males, the excess of testosterone leads to precocious puberty, with penile and muscle enlargement. In females, it can lead to masculinization before birth. Female fetuses exhibit clitoral enlargement and labial fusion. Genital ambiguity may be so profound that inappropriate sex assignment (**44**) is made at birth. There may be early growth of pubic hair and other pubertal features. Adolescence girls have impaired breast development. Reproductive abnormalities are common in women, particularly those with the classical salt-wasting even if treatment was instituted at birth. Labial fusion due to androgen excess *in utero* may leave the vaginal introitus inadequate for successful coitus, and surgical correction may be necessary.

Both girls and boys have an increase in linear growth but if not treated, their epiphyses close

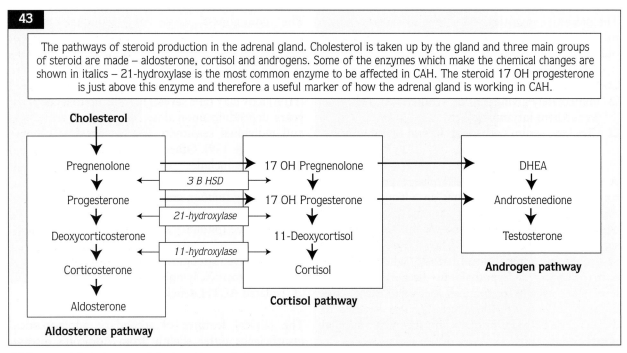

43

The pathways of steroid production in the adrenal gland. Cholesterol is taken up by the gland and three main groups of steroid are made – aldosterone, cortisol and androgens. Some of the enzymes which make the chemical changes are shown in italics – 21-hydroxylase is the most common enzyme to be affected in CAH. The steroid 17 OH progesterone is just above this enzyme and therefore a useful marker of how the adrenal gland is working in CAH.

43 Enzyme defects in congenital adrenal hyperplasia.

prematurely and their final height will be less than expected.

More than two-thirds of infants with 21-hydroxylase deficiency have the salt-wasting form of the disorder, with deficiency of both mineralocorticoid (aldosterone) and corticosteroid (cortisol) production. This condition presents early in life with hyponatraemia, hyperkalaemia, and hypotension.

Nonclassical (late-onset) CAH

Some girls or young women have no developmental abnormalities or salt-wasting, but have symptoms and signs of androgen excess at the time of puberty or soon thereafter. This has been referred to as nonclassical or late-onset 21-hydroxylase deficiency. It is manifested by hirsutism, acne, and menstrual irregularity in young women. These patients have sufficient aldosterone production and typically have the simple virilizing features.

Late-onset CAH may be suspected in a patient with elevated serum testosterone. However, the characteristic biochemical abnormality in patients with 21-hydroxylase deficiency is a high serum concentration of 17-hydroxyprogesterone (17-OHP), the normal substrate for the 21-hydroxylase enzyme. A morning 17-OHP >20 nmol/l suggests the diagnosis, which may be confirmed by a high dose 250 µg Synacthen test. The response to this ACTH injection is exaggerated, and most patients have 17-OHP levels exceeding 40 nmol/l. Patients with the salt-wasting form of 21-hydroxylase deficiency have low serum concentrations of aldosterone and 11-deoxycorticosterone, with increased plasma renin activity. Genetic testing to identify specific mutations is possible in >90% of those affected. It can be used to test other members of a family with a known predisposition.

ADRENAL GLAND MASSES – INCIDENTALOMAS

With the advent of technological advances in imaging, such as CT and MRI, incidental adrenal masses are more frequently being found. An adrenal incidentaloma is a mass lesion greater than 1 cm in diameter discovered by radiological examination. An adrenal lump may be found in up to 10% of the population at autopsy. There are two important questions to ask when an adrenal mass is picked up incidentally:
❏ Is it malignant?
❏ Is it functioning?

Adrenal malignancy may be primary or secondary. Primary adrenocortical carcinomas are significantly associated with mass size, with 90% being more than 4 cm in diameter when discovered, although a majority of masses larger than 4 cm in diameter are benign. MRI or CT with 3 or 5 mm cuts may allow prediction of the histologic type of the adrenal tumour, which is particularly important in the evaluation of masses that do not meet the size criterion for removal. The lipid-rich nature of cortical adenomas is helpful in distinguishing this benign tumour from carcinoma.

If an adrenal mass measured on an unenhanced CT has the density of fat, the likelihood that it is a benign adenoma is nearly 100%. A homogeneous adrenal mass with a smooth border and an attenuation value <10 HU on unenhanced CT is very likely to be a benign adenoma. Adrenal adenomas also show a much earlier washout of contrast enhancement than do nonadenomas. T1- and T2-weighted imaging on MRI scanning can help distinguish benign adenomas from malignancy and

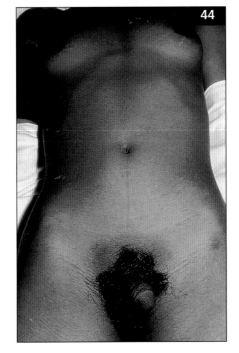

44 Congenital adrenal hyperplasia. Excessive virilization in a female raised as a male. (Courtesy of Manson Publishing: *Paediatrics and Child Health*, 2007.)

phaeochromocytoma. The following features suggest a benign adrenal tumour:

❑ Round and homogeneous density with smooth contour.
❑ Diameter less than 4 cm; unilateral location.
❑ Unilateral.
❑ Low unenhanced CT attenuation values.
❑ Limited enhancement on CT with intravenous contrast.
❑ Isointensity with liver on both T1- and T2-weighted MRI.

Adrenal cysts, hamatomas, and lipomas are usually easily characterized because of their distinctive imaging characteristics. Cytology from a specimen obtained by fine-needle aspiration (FNA) cannot distinguish a benign adrenal mass from the rare adrenal carcinoma. It can, however, distinguish between an adrenal tumour and a metastatic tumour. Thus, FNA is not useful in the routine evaluation of incidentalomas in patients suspected to have small nonadrenal cancers. Phaeochromocytoma should always be excluded with normal values of 24-hour urinary excretion of catecholamines before attempting FNA biopsy of an adrenal mass.

Fifteen percent of adrenal incidentalomas are functional hormone-secreting tumours. These include phaeochromocytoma, cortisol-, androgen-, and aldosterone-secreting tumours. The presence of a functioning mass is suspected by the history, e.g. palpitations, sweating, or headache, physical examination, e.g. features of Cushing's syndrome, androgenization, or hypertension, and routine laboratory findings (e.g. hypokalemia). Subclinical Cushing's syndrome and phaeochromocytoma are sufficiently common that all patients with an adrenal incidentaloma should be screened for these disorders. In addition, hypertensive patients should be screened for an aldosterone-secreting tumour even if the serum potassium concentration is normal.

PITUITARY DISEASE
PITUITARY HORMONE EXCESS
Hyperprolactinaemia
Hyperprolactinaemia is common and may be found in up to 25% of women with an irregular menstrual cycle. A raised serum prolactin (PRL) may be due to the influence of drug therapy or a range of physiological states, including most commonly polycystic ovarian syndrome (PCOS). Higher serum levels of PRL (>1000 mU/l) are most likely to be due to prolactinoma, a tumour of the pituitary gland. Other causes relate to decreased dopaminergic inhibition of PRL secretion or decreased clearance of PRL.

Serum PRL concentrations in patients who have prolactinomas can range from minimally elevated levels to exceedingly high (400–100 000 mU/l). With hyperprolactinemia due to other causes, the concentrations rarely exceed 3000 mU/l. Prolactinomas are the most frequent of the hormone-secreting pituitary adenomas, accounting for approximately 30–40% of all recognized pituitary adenomas. They are most common in women aged 20–40 years. Prolactinomas in men are usually larger, due to the lack of symptoms or delay in seeking medical attention. In men, they have a more rapid rate of growth. Most prolactinomas are sporadic but they can rarely occur as part of the Type 1 MEN syndrome. They are nearly always benign but, rarely, can be malignant and metastasize.

Several conditions interfere with normal dopamine inhibition of PRL secretion. This can be through damage to the dopaminergic neurones of the hypothalamus, sectioning of the pituitary stalk, or via drugs that block dopamine receptors on the pituitary gland. *Table 31* presents the causes of hyperprolactinaemia.

Table 31 Causes of hyperprolactinaemia

❑ Prolactinoma
❑ Tumours of the hypothalamus, both benign (e.g. craniopharyngiomas) and malignant (e.g. metastatic breast carcinoma)
❑ Infiltrative diseases of the hypothalamus (e.g. sarcoidosis)
❑ Section of the hypothalamic pituitary stalk (e.g. due to head trauma or surgery)
❑ Adenomas of the pituitary other than lactotroph adenomas
❑ Oestrogen-containing products
❑ Hypothyroidism (increased TRH and pituitary response to TRH)
❑ Chest wall injury
❑ Chronic renal failure
❑ Pregnancy
❑ Stress
❑ Nipple stimulation
❑ Drug treatments

Drugs are commonly implicated as a cause of raised serum PRL and it is essential to take a careful drug history. Commonly used drugs that are implicated in hyperprolactinaemia include:

- ❏ Phenothiazines.
- ❏ Haloperidol.
- ❏ Risperidone.
- ❏ Metoclopramide.
- ❏ Sulpiride.
- ❏ Cimetidine.
- ❏ Verapamil.
- ❏ Methyldopa.

Idiopathic hyperprolactinaemia

In a number of patients whose serum PRL concentration is between 400 and 1500 mU/l, no cause can be found. Although many of these patients may have microadenomas not visible on imaging studies, in most cases the serum PRL concentrations change little during follow-up.

Macroprolactinaemia

The most common form of PRL in serum is not glycosylated, but a small amount of 25-glycosylated form can also be detected. In rare cases, glycosylated PRL, which appears to circulate in aggregates, accounts for most serum PRL. This is seen in macroprolactinaemia. This is a benign clinical condition.

Hyperprolactinaemia in premenopausal women causes hypogonadism manifested by infertility, oligomenorrhoea or amenorrhoea, and galactorrhoea.

Excluding pregnancy, hyperprolactinaemia accounts for approximately 10–20% of cases of amenorrhoea. The mechanism involves inhibition of luteinizing hormone (LH) and follicle stimulating hormone (FSH) secretion, via inhibition of the release of gonadotrophin releasing hormone (GnRH). The symptoms of hypogonadism due to hyperprolactinaemia in premenopausal women correlate with the magnitude of the hyperprolactinaemia.

Hypogonadism is typically associated with subnormal oestroegen secretion leading to oligomenorrhoea, amenorrhoea, subfertlility, hot flushes, and vaginal dryness. Hyperprolactinaemia in premenopausal women frequently leads to galactorrhoea.

Women with amenorrhoea secondary to hyperprolactinaemia have a lower spine and forearm bone mineral density compared with normal women or women with hyperprolactinaemia and normal menses. In postmenopausal women, galactorrhoea is rare. Hyperprolactinaemia in these women may only be recognized if a prolactinoma causes headaches or impairs vision (see later).

In men, hyperprolactinaemia also causes hypogonadotropic hypogonadism, leading to decreased libido, impotence, infertility, gynaecomastia and, rarely, galactorrhoea. There is a correlation between the presence of these symptoms and the degree of hyperprolactinaemia. Hyperprolactinaemia causes decreased testosterone concentrations that are not associated with an increase in LH secretion. In the long-term there may be symptoms of decreased muscle mass, body hair, erectile dysfunction, and osteoporosis. Infertility is occasionally seen.

As part of a detailed history one should inquire about pregnancy, medications that can cause hyperprolactinaemia, headache, visual symptoms, symptoms of hypothyroidism, and a history of renal disease. The physical examination should be directed toward testing for a local compressive features (e.g. bitemporal field loss), and examining for signs of hypothyroidism or hypogonadism.

Investigations for hyperprolactinaemia

Women with oligomenorrhoea, amenorrhoea, or galactorrhoea and men with symptoms of hypogonadism or impotence or infertility should have their serum PRL measured. The usual normal range for serum PRL is 80–400 mU/l. Serum PRL concentrations may increase slightly during sleep, strenuous exercise, emotional or physical stress, intense breast stimulation, and high-protein meals.

The PRL concentration tends to vary with the size of the adenoma. Adenomas less than 1 cm diameter are typically associated with serum PRL values below 3000 mU/l and those greater than 2.0 cm in diameter with values above 15 000 mU/l. This may not be true with a largely cystic tumour. Occasionally, a discrepancy between the large size of an adenoma and modest elevation of the PRL concentration is due to an artefact in the immunoradiometric assay for PRL. This artefact, called the 'hook effect', can be obviated by dilution of the sera, which will allow a true assessment of the PRL concentration.

Tests for thyroid and renal function should be carried out. MRI of the pituitary gland should be performed in a patient with any degree of hyperprolactinaemia to look for a mass lesion in the hypothalamic–pituitary region. If there is a mass in the region of the hypothalamus or pituitary then a full pituitary hormone profile should be carried out.

Galactorrhoea without hyperprolactinaemia

The serum PRL concentration is often normal in women who present with galactorrhoea. Galactorrhoea in the absence of hyperprolactinaemia does not need to be treated unless symptoms are disturbing for the patient.

Acromegaly

Acromegaly is the clinical syndrome that results from excessive secretion of growth hormone (GH). The annual incidence is three per million of the population. The mean age at diagnosis is 40–45 years. GH excess that occurs before fusion of the epiphyseal growth plates in a child or adolescent is called pituitary gigantism. GH excess that occurs after fusion of the epiphyseal growth plates is called acromegaly.

The most common cause of acromegaly is a pituitary (GH-secreting) adenoma of the anterior pituitary. These adenomas account for about one-third of all hormone-secreting pituitary adenomas. The other rare causes of acromegaly include excess secretion of growth hormone releasing hormone (GHRH) by hypothalamic tumours, ectopic GHRH secretion by nonendocrine tumours such as carcinoid tumours or small-cell lung cancers, and ectopic secretion of GH by nonendocrine tumours.

The clinical features of acromegaly are attributable to high serum concentrations of both GH and insulin-like growth factor-1 (IGF-1), a GH-stimulated hormone produced in the liver. These hormones stimulate the growth of many tissues, such as skin, connective tissue, cartilage, bone, viscera, and many epithelia. In addition, the pituitary adenoma may cause local symptoms such as headache (60%), visual field defects (classically bitemporal hemianopsia), and cranial nerve palsies.

Clinical features of GH excess

The interval from the onset of symptoms until diagnosis is about 12 years. At diagnosis, about 75% of patients have macroadenomas (a tumour diameter of 1 cm or greater), and some of the adenomas extend to the parasellar or suprasellar regions. Patients with acromegaly have a number of characteristic physical features (**45**):

❏ Acral overgrowth (**46a**). The characteristic findings are an enlarged jaw (macrognathia) and enlarged, swollen hands (**46b**) and feet. These result in increasing shoe and glove size and the need to enlarge rings. The facial features become

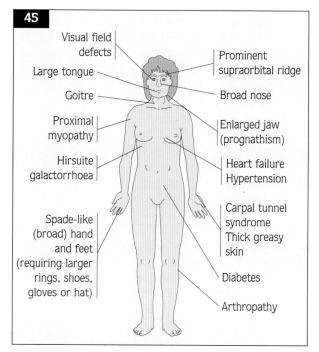

45 Diagram to illustrate the characteristics of the acromegalic patient.

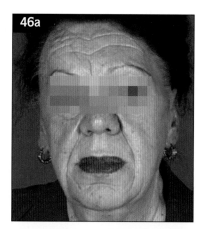

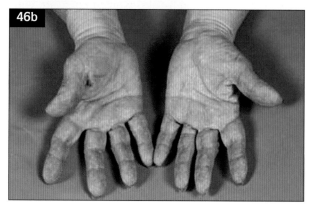

46 (**a**) Typical facies in an acromegaly patient. (**b**) Palms in a patient with acromegaly. (Courtesy of Dr J. Thomas, St Bartholomew's Hospital, London.)

coarse, with enlargement of the nose and frontal bones as well as the jaw, and the teeth become spread apart.

❏ Articular overgrowth. Synovial tissue and cartilage also enlarge, causing hypertrophic arthropathy of the knees, ankles, hips, spine, and other joints. Joint symptoms are a common presenting feature of the disease.

❏ Cardiovascular disease. Cardiovascular abnormalities include hypertension, left ventricular hypertrophy, and cardiomyopathy. The cardiomyopathy is characterized by diastolic dysfunction and arrhythmias. Heart failure occurs in 5% of patients. An increased prevalence of valvular heart disease has also been reported.

❏ Pituitary dysfunction. A macroadenoma can cause decreased secretion of other pituitary hormones, most commonly gonadotrophins. Many women with acromegaly have menstrual dysfunction, with or without galactorrhoea, and some have hot flushes and vaginal atrophy. Men may have erectile dysfunction, loss of libido, decreased facial hair growth, and testicular atrophy.

❏ The hypogonadism is caused either by the mass effect of the pituitary tumour or by hyperprolactinaemia (present in about 30% of patients). Hypothyroidism and hypoadrenalism occur less commonly.

❏ Skin and hair changes. The skin thickens, making it hard to puncture, and skin tags may appear. Hyperhidrosis is common, often making the patient malodorous. Hair growth increases, and some women have hirsutism.

❏ Soft tissues. Manifestations of soft tissue overgrowth include macroglossia, deepening of the voice, and paraesthesias of the hands (e.g. carpal tunnel syndrome in 20%). Macroglossia and enlargement of the soft tissues of the pharynx and larynx can lead to obstructive sleep apnoea.

❏ Tumours. Acromegaly is associated with an increased risk of uterine leiomyomata and colonic polyps. Some studies have reported premalignant adenomatous colonic polyps in up to 30% of patients.

❏ Viscera. Many visceral organs are enlarged in acromegaly, including the thyroid, heart, liver, kidneys, and prostate. The thyroid enlargement may be diffuse or multinodular. Thyroid function is usually normal in these patients. Reversible prostatic enlargement is common.

❏ Diabetes. Overt diabetes occurs in 10–15% of cases. Impaired glucose tolerance occurs in >50%.

❏ Other. Fatigue and weakness are commonly reported.

The mortality rate of patients with acromegaly is two to three times the expected rate, mostly from cardiovascular diseases and malignancy. Death rate is significantly correlated with higher serum GH concentrations and the presence at diagnosis of cardiovascular disease, hypertension, or diabetes mellitus. If treatment lowers the serum GH concentration to normal, outcomes are much improved.

Investigations for acromegaly
Both serum GH concentrations and IGF-1 concentrations are increased in virtually all patients with acromegaly. Some patients have hyper-triglyceridaemia or hypercalciuria. Most patients have raised serum concentrations of phosphate due to a direct stimulation of renal tubular phosphate reabsorption by IGF-1. Hyperprolactinaemia occurs in about 30% of patients. In some patients it is due to co-secretion of PRL and GH by a somato-mammotroph adenoma, and levels may be very high. In other patients the cause is likely interference with hypothalamic–pituitary blood flow, in which cases the serum PRL concentration will be less than 3000 mU/l. The secretion of other pituitary hormones, most often gonadotrophins, may be decreased in patients with macroadenomas.

Once a patient is suspected to have acromegaly the diagnosis can be confirmed by measurement of both serum GH concentration after a glucose load and GH-dependent circulating molecules, such as IGF-1 and insulin-like growth factor binding protein-3 (IGFBP-3).

❏ Serum IGF-1 concentration. Unlike growth hormone, serum IGF-1 concentrations do not vary from hour to hour according to food intake, exercise or sleep, but instead reflect integrated GH secretion during the preceding day or longer. Serum IGF-1 concentrations are elevated in virtually all patients with acromegaly. The results must be interpreted, however, according to the patient's age. In normal subjects, serum IGF-1 concentrations are highest during puberty and decline gradually thereafter.

❑ Serum GH concentration. Serum GH concentrations may be elevated but can also be high in patients with uncontrolled diabetes mellitus, liver disease, and malnutrition. All patients with acromegaly have increased GH secretion. However, the random serum GH concentration is often in the range of 10–30 mU/l, a value that can be found in normal subjects. In acromegaly, the serum GH changes little during the day or night or in response to stimuli such as food or exercise.

❑ Oral glucose tolerance test (OGTT). This is the most specific dynamic test for establishing the diagnosis of acromegaly. In normal subjects, serum GH concentrations fall to <5 mU/l (1 ng/ml) or less within 2 hours after ingestion of 75 g glucose. Levels greater than 10 mU/l are found in more than 85% of patients with acromegaly. If one of the newer, highly sensitive immunoradiometric or immunochemiluminescent GH assays is used, there may be a greater reduction in serum GH concentration after oral glucose administration in normal subjects.

❑ IGFBP-3. IGFBP-3 is a binding protein, the secretion of which is GH dependent. Concentrations in serum are elevated in patients with acromegaly. There is, however, considerable overlap of these values with those in normal persons, limiting the utility of this measurement.

Once GH hypersecretion has been confirmed, MRI scanning of the pituitary should be performed. Pituitary tumours as small as 2 mm in diameter can be detected with this technique, and the dimensions and anatomic extent of the tumour can be accurately identified. CT is less sensitive. In 75% of patients the tumour is a macroadenoma (>10 mm). The tumour may extend to the parasellar or suprasellar region. Although not recommended for the diagnosis of acromegaly, a plain radiograph of the skull can show a number of features of acromegaly. In addition to the enlargement of the sella turcica, other changes that may be seen include elongation of the mandible, enlargement of the frontal and maxillary sinuses, and thickening of the cranial vault.

Other causes of acromegaly
Rare causes of acromegaly include pituitary somatotroph carcinoma, hypothalamic tumour secreting GHRH, nonendocrine tumour secreting GHRH, ectopic secretion of GH by a nonendocrine tumour, and excess growth factor activity. If the MRI of pituitary gland is normal, abdominal and chest imaging should be performed, followed by catheterization studies in an attempt to demonstrate an arteriovenous gradient of either GH or GHRH in the region of the tumour.

Ectopic GHRH secretion accounts for only 0.5% of cases of acromegaly. Serum GHRH is the only specific marker for this disorder and concentrations are usually elevated. Other conditions are described elsewhere: ACTH-secreting adenoma – see Adrenal hormone excess (page 60); TSH-secreting adenoma – see Thyrotoxicosis (page 49); syndrome of inappropriate antidiuretic hormone (SIADH) – see Electrolyte disturbances and hyponatraemia (page 85).

SELLAR MASSES

There is a range of lesions that can involve the sellar region that is inhabited by the pituitary gland.

Pituitary adenomas

These are the most common cause of sellar masses in adulthood, accounting for up to 10% of all intracranial neoplasms. Other disorders, which are often difficult to distinguish from pituitary adenomas by imaging, include benign and malignant tumours. Nonfunctioning pituitary adenomas are tumours of the anterior pituitary that are almost always benign. They may be seen as part of Type 1 MEN syndrome.

Adenomas are classified by their size and the cell of origin. Lesions smaller than 1 cm are classified as microadenomas, and lesions larger than 1 cm are classified as macroadenomas. These tumours can arise from any type of cell of the anterior pituitary and may result in increased secretion of the hormone(s) produced by that cell and/or decreased secretion of other hormones due to compression of other cell types. Tumours include:

❑ Gonadotrophinomas. These are the most common pituitary macroadenomas but secrete inefficiently and variably. They rarely cause symptoms and are the most common clinically nonfunctioning pituitary adenomas.

❑ Thyrotrophinomas. These may present as clinically nonfunctioning sellar masses; they may cause hyperthyroidism due to increased secretion of intact TSH.

❑ Prolactinomas. These usually cause hyperprolactinaemia, which leads to hypogonadism in women and men.

❑ Somatotrophinomas. These typically cause acromegaly due to increased GH secretion.

❑ Corticotrophinomas. These usually cause Cushing's disease (see page 61).

Craniopharyngioma

These are solid or mixed solid–cystic benign tumours that arise from remnants of Rathke's pouch along a line from the nasopharynx to the diencephalon. Most are either intrasellar or suprasellar. About 50% present clinically during childhood and adolescence, the other 50% present after age 20 years. The major presenting symptoms are growth retardation in children and abnormal vision in adults. In addition, pituitary hormonal deficiencies, including diabetes insipidus, are common.

Meningioma

This is a typically benign tumour arising from the meninges. Some arise near the sella, causing visual impairment and hormonal deficiencies.

Malignant tumours

Some malignant tumours arise within or near the sella, and others metastasize to this site. Primary malignancies that arise in the parasellar region include germ cell tumours, sarcomas, chordomas, and lymphomas. Pituitary carcinomas are rare.

Germ cell tumours usually occur through the third decade of life and may present with headache, nausea, vomiting, lethargy, diplopia, hypopituitarism, or diabetes insipidus (with suprasellar tumours), and paralysis of upward conjugate gaze. A mass in the third ventricle is seen by imaging. They are highly radiosensitive.

Chordomas are locally aggressive tumours that can metastasize. They present with headaches, visual impairment, and anterior pituitary hormonal deficiencies.

Primary central nervous system lymphomas can sometimes involve the pituitary and hypothalamus. Metastases to the hypothalamus and pituitary gland account for 1–2% of sellar masses. They occur most commonly with breast cancer in women and lung cancer in men. Symptoms include diabetes insipidus, anterior pituitary dysfunction, visual field defects, retroorbital pain, and ophthalmoplegia.

Other masses include cysts, abscesses, and fistula. Rathke's cleft, arachnoid, and dermoid cysts can produce sellar enlargement resulting in visual impairment, diabetes insipidus, anterior pituitary hormonal deficiencies, and hydrocephalus. Pituitary abcesses are rare with most patients diagnosed at the time of surgical exploration.

Arteriovenous fistula of the cavernous sinus can cause enlargement of the pituitary gland.

Common presenting features of a pituitary adenoma
Gonadotroph and other clinically nonfunctioning adenomas usually come to clinical attention when they become large enough to cause neurological symptoms. They may also be recognized when an imaging procedure of the head is performed for an unrelated reason or, uncommonly, because of hormonal hypersecretion. Neurological symptoms include:

❑ Impaired vision. This is the most common symptom that leads a patient with a clinically nonfunctioning adenoma to seek medical attention. Visual impairment is caused by suprasellar extension of the adenoma that compresses the optic chiasm. The most common complaint is diminished vision in the temporal fields (bitemporal hemianopia). One or both eyes may be affected, and, if both, to variable degrees. Diminished visual acuity occurs when the optic chiasm is more severely compressed. Other patterns of visual loss may also occur. Thus, an intrasellar lesion should be suspected when there is any unexplained pattern of visual loss.

❑ Headaches, caused by expansion of the sella. The quality of the headache is nonspecific.

❑ Diplopia. This may be induced by oculomotor nerve compression resulting from lateral extension of the adenoma.

❑ Cerebrospinal fluid rhinorrhoea, caused by inferior extension of the adenoma.

❑ Pituitary apoplexy, induced by sudden haemorrhage into the adenoma, causing excruciating headache and diplopia.

Symptoms due to excess gonadotrophins are rare, but ovarian hyperstimulation in premenopausal women and, rarely, in prepubertal girls can occur due to excess gonadotrophin secretion. Premenopausal women present with amenorrhoea or oligomenorrhoea. In men, elevated serum concentrations of testosterone may be seen due to hypersecretion of intact LH. Abnormalities in children can lead to premature puberty.

Investigations of sellar masses
MRI is the best imaging procedure for most sellar masses. A mass that is separate from the pituitary gland generally indicates that the mass is not a pituitary adenoma.

Current imaging techniques are sufficiently sensitive to detect any pituitary adenoma that has become so large as to impair vision or cause any other neurological symptom, or one which causes hormonal abnormalities. MRI scanning may not distinguish adenomatous tissue from normal pituitary tissue. Normal pituitary tissue and most sellar lesions, pituitary adenomas, and other tumours, have a signal that is similar to or slightly greater in intensity than that of central nervous system tissue.

Cystic lesions, such as Rathke's cleft cysts, often have a low intensity signal on T1-weighted images; however, craniopharyngiomas and even pituitary adenomas may be partially cystic and, therefore, have low intensity signals. Meningiomas typically have a brighter and more homogeneous signal than pituitary adenomas. They also have a suprasellar rather than a sellar centre and an attachment to the dura may be seen after contrast enhancement.

Gadolinium-enhanced imaging can be used. Normal pituitary tissue takes up gadolinium to a greater degree than central nervous system (CNS) tissue and, therefore, has a higher intensity signal than the surrounding CNS. Both micro- and macroadenomas of the pituitary (as well as other sellar masses such as craniopharyngiomas and meningiomas) usually take up gadolinium to a lesser degree than the normal pituitary but more than the surrounding tissue.

Any patient with an intrasellar mass detected by MRI should be evaluated further by measurement of serum concentrations of pituitary hormones to determine if the lesion is of pituitary or nonpituitary origin. This includes a serum PRL, thyroid function tests, IGF-1, and a screening test for Cushing's syndrome. The patient should be clinically assessed for acromegaly, Cushing's syndrome, and hypopituitarism in addition to a visual assessment (fundoscopy and visual fields). Recognizing the gonadotroph origin of an intrasellar mass is more difficult. Basal serum concentrations of intact FSH and LH in women give the appearance of the menopause or premature ovarian failure. However, a markedly supranormal FSH level with a subnormal LH concentration, or a markedly elevated serum oestradiol with an FSH concentration that is not suppressed, suggest a functioning gonadotrophinoma. In men, a supranormal serum LH accompanied by a supranormal serum testosterone is strong evidence that the lesion is one of the unusual gonadotroph adenomas that secretes intact LH.

Hormonal hyposecretion can be caused by almost any hypothalamic or pituitary lesion. An exception is central diabetes insipidus since this indicates that the lesion affects the hypothalamus or the pituitary stalk rather than the pituitary gland itself.

No evaluation for hormonal hyposecretion or visual abnormalities is necessary in the patient with a microadenoma of the pituitary gland.

PITUITARY HORMONE DEFICIENCY

Hypopituitarism refers to a decreased secretion of pituitary hormones, which can result from disease of the pituitary gland itself or the hypothalamus with diminished secretion of hypothalamic releasing hormones. Causes are listed in *Table 32*.

Lymphocytic hypophysitis is an uncommon disorder that is initially characterized by lymphocytic infiltration and enlargement of the pituitary, followed by destruction of the pituitary cells. It most often occurs in late pregnancy or the postpartum period and is more common in women. Affected patients typically present with severe headache and hypopituitarism. MRI typically reveals features of a pituitary mass, but enhancement may be delayed or even absent in the posterior pituitary area. The natural history typically involves progressive pituitary atrophy with replacement of pituitary tissue by fibrosis. High-dose pulse glucocorticoid therapy has been reported to reduce the mass effect in a number of patients.

Infarction of the pituitary gland after substantial blood loss during childbirth has long been recognized as a cause of hypopituitarism and is called Sheehan's syndrome. Severe hypopituitarism can be recognized during the first days or weeks after delivery by the development of lethargy, anorexia, weight loss, and inability to lactate. Another rare cause of pituitary infarction in older patients is vascular insufficiency occurring during coronary artery bypass surgery.

Sudden haemorrhage into the pituitary gland is called pituitary apoplexy. Haemorrhage often occurs into a pituitary adenoma. Apoplexy can present with sudden onset of severe headache, diplopia due to pressure on the oculomotor nerves, and hypopituitarism. The sudden onset of ACTH deficiency can cause life-threatening hypotension. The hypopituitarism and visual disturbance may improve after surgical decompression of the pituitary. This is the recommended early therapy. Both problems may also improve spontaneously, as blood is resorbed, over a course of weeks to months after the haemorrhage.

Mutations in the PROP-1 gene appear to be the most common causes of both familial and sporadic congenital combined pituitary hormone deficiency, including deficiencies of GH, PRL, TSH, LH, and FSH. GH deficiency is the most common isolated pituitary hormone deficiency. It usually begins in infancy or childhood and results in short stature.

An empty sella refers to an enlarged sella turcica that is not entirely filled with pituitary tissue. This can occur as a result of treatment, typically surgery or radiotherapy. There may also be a primary defect in the diaphragma sella that leads to cerebrospinal fluid (CSF) enlarging the sella region. Primary defects are not typically associated with hormone deficiencies.

Diseases of the hypothalamus can affect anterior hormone secretion and also diminish the secretion of ADH, resulting in diabetes insipidus. Benign tumours may arise in the hypothalamus (e.g. craniopharyngioma) and malignant tumours may metastasize here, e.g. lung and breast carcinoma. Infiltrative disorders such as sarcoidosis and Langerhans cell histiocytosis can cause deficiencies of anterior pituitary hormones and diabetes insipidus. Head trauma of sufficient severity to fracture the skull base can cause hypothalamic hormone deficiencies, resulting in deficient secretion of anterior pituitary hormones and ADH.

Table 32 Causes of pituitary hormone deficiency

- ❑ Pituitary tumour
- ❑ Other sellar tumours (craniopharyngioma, meningioma, metastatic deposits, chordoma, glioma)
- ❑ Surgical hypophysectomy
- ❑ Radiotherapy (cranial, pituitary, nasopharyngeal)
- ❑ Infarction (pituitary apoplexy, Sheehan's syndrome)
- ❑ Empty sella
- ❑ Tuberculosis
- ❑ Trauma
- ❑ Infiltrative diseae (sarcoid, lymphocytic hypophysitis, haemachromatosis, histiocytosis X)
- ❑ Isolated hormone deficiencies (e.g. Kallman's syndrome [GnRH deficiency])

Clinical features of hypopituitarism

The presentation of hypopituitarism can be considered as the presentation of deficiency of each anterior pituitary hormone, local compressive effects of the tumour (headache, visual disturbance – see Sellar masses, page 74), and effects that relate to the underlying disease process (e.g. metastatic disease or sarcoid).

The presentation of patients with deficiencies of these hormones is often similar to that of patients with primary deficiencies of the target gland hormones they control.

Symptoms depend on the rate of onset and amount of hormone deficiency. Some diseases affect anterior pituitary cells suddenly, such as pituitary apoplexy. Other insults, such as radiation therapy to the pituitary or hypothalamus, usually act slowly, causing symptoms many years later. The severity of the hormonal deficiency is important. Complete ACTH and cortisol deficiency can cause symptoms under basal circumstances, while partial ACTH deficiency may cause symptoms only during times of physical stress.

If all the pituitary hormones are reduced, this is called panhypopituitarism. As a general rule, the secretion of gonadotrophins and GH is more likely to be affected than ACTH and TSH, but one cannot make an assumption about the status of one pituitary hormone from the status of another hormone.

ACTH deficiency

The absence of ACTH can lead to death due to vascular collapse, since cortisol is necessary for maintenance of peripheral vascular tone. A less severe form of the same phenomenon is postural hypotension and tachycardia. Mild, chronic deficiency may result in lassitude, fatigue, anorexia, weight loss, decreased libido, hypoglycaemia, and eosinophilia.

> *Unlike adrenal insufficiency (Addison's disease), primary ACTH deficiency does not cause salt-wasting, volume contraction, hyperpigmentation, or hyperkalaemia, because it does not result in a clinically important deficiency of aldosterone. Both forms of adrenal insufficiency can cause hyponatremia.*

Moderately severe ACTH and cortisol deficiency may cause few or no symptoms and no physical findings. Consequently, the adequacy of ACTH secretion should be evaluated biochemically in all patients who have pituitary or hypothalamic disease.

TSH deficiency

The clinical presentation of TSH deficiency is that of thyroxine deficiency, which might include fatigue, lethargy, cold intolerance, decreased appetite, constipation, facial puffiness, dry skin, bradycardia, delayed relaxation phase of the deep tendon reflexes, and anaemia. The degree of symptoms and abnormal physical findings usually parallels the degree of thyroxine deficiency. Some patients with marked TSH deficiency have few or no symptoms.

Gonadotrophin deficiency

Deficient secretion of the gonadotrophins FSH and LH causes hypogonadism in both women and men. In women, hypogonadism results in the inability to ovulate, infertility, and decreased oestrogen secretion. This can cause oligo- or amenorrhoea, vaginal dryness and atrophy, hot flushes, and fatigue. Subsequently breast tissue decreases, fine facial wrinkles appear, and bone mineral density declines. In men, hypogonadism means testicular hypofunction, which results in infertility and decreased testosterone secretion. This can lead to decreased muscle mass, decreased bone mineral density, and other features of hypogonadism (see Male hypogonadism, page 92).

GH deficiency

GH deficiency in children typically presents as short stature. GH deficiency in adults is linked to the following features:
❏ Diminished muscle mass and increased fat mass. This effect is the best documented.
❏ Increased serum LDL-cholesterol.
❏ Decreased bone mineral density.
❏ Diminished sense of well being.
❏ Increased risk of cardiovascular disease and increased inflammatory cardiovascular risk.

PRL deficiency

The only known presentation of PRL deficiency is the inability to lactate after delivery.

Diagnosing hypopituitarism

Hypopituitarism is defined as deficient secretion of one or more pituitary hormones because of pituitary or hypothalamic disease. To diagnose the condition each pituitary hormone may need to be tested separately, since there is a variable pattern of hormone deficiency among patients with hypopituitarism. In addition to determining hormone deficiencies, MRI imaging of the pituitary is usually required to help elucidate the underlying cause and local extent of disease.

Diagnosing ACTH deficiency

The basal secretion of ACTH must be sufficient to maintain the serum cortisol concentration within the normal range. For survival, it must increase to raise serum cortisol concentrations in times of physical stress. To determine basal ACTH secretion, serum cortisol should be measured between 8 and 9 am, and the results should be interpreted as follows:
❏ A serum cortisol value of <100 nmol/l confirmed by a second determination, is strong evidence of cortisol deficiency. If there is no obvious cause for hypopituitarism, serum ACTH should be measured. A serum ACTH value not higher than normal is inappropriately low and establishes the diagnosis of secondary adrenal deficiency (i.e. pituitary or hypothalamic disease). A value higher than normal indicates primary adrenal insufficiency (i.e. adrenal disease – see Adrenal hormone deficiency, page 64).
❏ A serum cortisol value >500 nmol/l indicates that basal ACTH secretion is sufficient, and also that it is probably sufficient for times of physical stress.
❏ A serum cortisol value of 100–500 nmol/l on two occasions is an indication to evaluate ACTH reserve.

Insulin tolerance test

Test of ACTH reserve uses the insulin-induced hypoglycaemia test (insulin tolerance test [ITT]). Hypoglycaemia is a sufficient stress to stimulate ACTH and therefore cortisol secretion. The test is performed by administering 0.1 unit of insulin per kg of body weight intravenously, and measuring serum glucose and serum cortisol before and 15, 30, 60, 90 and 120 minutes after the injection. In normal subjects, serum cortisol increases to 500 nmol/l if the serum glucose falls to 2.8 mmol/l.

This test can be dangerous in elderly patients and those with cardiovascular or cerebrovascular disease or epilepsy. Close monitoring is necessary to detect neuroglycopenic symptoms, which should be treated with intravenous glucose.

Hypoglycaemia induced by glucagon administration is sometimes used but is less reliable than the ITT.

Short synacthen test

Adrenal glands tend to atrophy when they have not been stimulated for a prolonged period, and do not secrete cortisol normally in response to a bolus dose of synacthen (synthetic ACTH). A serum cortisol concentration of 500 nmol/l) is considered a normal response. A patient with partial ACTH deficiency may respond normally to this test.

Metyrapone test

Metyrapone blocks 11-beta-hydroxylase (CYP11B1), the enzyme that catalyses the conversion of 11-deoxycortisol to cortisol. If the HPA axis is normal, there is a decline in serum cortisol with an increase in ACTH secretion and, therefore, an increase in 11-deoxycortisol. In normal subjects, administration of 750 mg of metyrapone orally every 4 hours for 24 hours results in a decline in 8 am serum cortisol to less than 172 nmol/l and an elevation in 8 am serum 11-deoxycortisol to 300 nmol/l at 24 hours. In patients who have decreased ACTH reserve due to hypothalamic or pituitary disease, the serum 11-deoxycortisol concentration will be less than 300 nmol/l at 24 hours. For this test to be considered reliable there should be a reduction in serum cortisol (<200 nmol/l).

Diagnosing TSH deficiency

In a patient with known hypothalamic or pituitary disease, the adequacy of TSH secretion can be assessed simply by measuring free circulating thyroxine (T4). If the serum T4 concentration is normal, TSH secretion is normal; if the serum T4 concentration is low, TSH secretion is low.

In patients who have hypothyroidism due to damage to the hypothalamus or pituitary, the serum TSH concentration is usually not helpful in making the diagnosis of hypothyroidism, because a low serum T4 concentration is usually associated with a serum TSH concentration within the normal range. Serum TSH alone should not be used as a screening test for hypothyroidism in patients who have pituitary or hypothalamic disease. It is also an unreliable measurement in patients who are acutely unwell. Where there remains doubt about TSH reserve, a TRH test can be performed.

TRH is administered intravenously (0.2 mg) and T4 and TSH are measured at 0, 20, and 60 minutes. With pituitary TSH deficiency, the TSH will fail to rise in response to TRH. In hypothalamic disease, there is a rise but it is delayed until 60 minutes instead of the normal response which is to peak at 20 minutes.

Diagnosing gonadotrophin (LH/FSH) deficiency

In men, LH deficiency can best be detected by measurement of the serum testosterone. If it is repeatedly low at 8–10 am, LH secretion is subnormal and the patient has secondary hypogonadism. When the serum testosterone concentration is low, the serum LH concentration is usually within the normal range, but low compared to elevated values in primary hypogonadism. If fertility is an issue, the sperm count should be determined.

In women of premenopausal age, if the patient has pituitary or hypothalamic disease with normal menstruation then no tests of LH or FSH are required since there is intact pituitary–gonadal function. If the woman has oligomenorrhoea or amenorrhoea, serum oestrogen and LH or FSH should be measured. If oestradiol levels are low with no elevation of gonadotrophins this is suggestive of gonadotrophin deficiency. This can be confirmed with GnRH test. Serum LH response to a single bolus dose of GnRH may be subnormal, suggesting diminished gonadotrophin reserve.

In women of postmenopausal age, gonadotrophin levels are normally elevated. Low levels are diagnostic of gonadotrophin deficiency.

Diagnosing GH deficiency

Measurement of basal serum GH concentration does not distinguish reliably between normal and subnormal GH secretion in adults. However, the likelihood that the GH response to all provocative stimuli will be subnormal in patients who have an organic pituitary diseases plus deficiencies of ACTH, TSH, and gonadotrophins is about 95%.

A serum IGF-1 concentration lower than the age-specific lower limit of normal in a patient who has organic pituitary disease confirms the diagnosis of GH deficiency. Provocative tests of GH secretion include insulin-induced hypoglycaemia or the combination of arginine and GHRH. Subnormal increases in the serum GH concentration in a patient who has organic pituitary disease confirms the diagnosis of GH deficiency. Other stimulation tests have been used, including arginine alone, clonidine, L-DOPA, and the combination of arginine and L-DOPA; however, these are more likely to give false positive results.

Diagnosing PRL deficiency
There is no standardized test of PRL reserve. It is not necessary since there is no available treatment option.

ADH deficiency – diabetes insipidus (DI)
The characteristic presenting feature of DI is the passage of large volumes (>3 l/day in adults) of dilute urine (osmolarity <300 mOsmol/l). Characteristic symptoms are polyuria, nocturia, and thirst. There are three major causes of this clinical and biochemical presentation:
❑ Cranial DI is associated with deficient secretion of ADH. It is most commonly idiopathic but can be induced by trauma and pituitary/hypothalamic disease.
❑ Nephrogenic DI is characterized by normal ADH secretion with varying degrees of renal resistance to its water-retaining effect.
❑ Compulsive water drinking (primary polydipsia).

The patient should be asked about the rate of onset of the polyuria. In adults, the onset is usually abrupt in cranial DI and gradual in acquired nephrogenic DI or primary polydipsia. There are familial forms of both cranial and nephrogenic DI. The defects in these disorders are due to mutations that impair either ADH synthesis or the renal response to ADH. Causes of DI are presented in *Table 33*.

Diagnosing DI
Screening tests should include confirmation of a large urine output (>3 l/day). A serum calcium, glucose, electrolytes, and creatinine will help to exclude a number of unrelated causes for polyuria. The definite investigation, however, is the fluid deprivation test.

In adults, the fluid deprivation test for the evaluation of polyuria involves measurement of the urine volume and osmolality every hour, and plasma sodium concentration and osmolality every 2 hours. Weight and vital signs are obtained every 2 hours for the first 4 hours and then hourly. This test should be carried out in the morning. The patient should avoid drinking for 3 hours prior to the onset of the test and is not allowed to drink during the test. In mild cases overnight water deprivation is suggested. However, severe volume depletion and hypernatraemia can be induced in patients with marked polyuria. The fluid deprivation test in adults is continued until one of the following occurs:
❑ The urine osmolality reaches a clearly normal value (above 600 mOsmol/l), indicating that both ADH release and effect are intact. Patients with partial DI may have a substantial rise in urine osmolality, but not to this extent.
❑ The patient has lost 5% of body weight or exhibits signs of volume depletion.
❑ The urine osmolality is stable on two or three successive measurements despite a rising plasma osmolality.
❑ The plasma osmolality exceeds 295–300 mOsmol/l.
❑ In the final two settings, exogenous ADH is then administered, 2 µg of desmopressin (DDAVP) intramuscularly and the urine osmolality and volume monitored, with measurement of the urine osmolality at baseline and at 30 minute intervals over the next 2 hours. In DI, if the urine osmolality does not increase by more than 100 mOsmol/l over baseline following the administration of DDAVP, the diagnosis of nephrogenic DI is made. A specimen should also be obtained for measurement of plasma ADH, which is always elevated during short dehydration tests in patients with hereditary nephrogenic DI.

Table 33 Causes of diabetes insipidus

Cranial
❑ Idiopathic
❑ Trauma (head injury/neurosurgery)
❑ Tumours (craniopharyngioma, metastatic disease
❑ Meningitis
❑ Infarction (e.g. Sheehan's syndrome)
❑ Meningitis
❑ Infiltrative conditions (sarcoid, tuberculosis, lymphocytic hypophysitis)
❑ Familial (autosomal dominant)
❑ DIDMOAD syndrome (diabetes insipidus, diabetes mellitus, optic atrophy, deafness)

Nephrogenic
❑ Familial
❑ Drugs (lithium, demeclocycline)
❑ Metabolic (hypercalcaemia, hyperglycaemia, hypokalaemia)
❑ Renal failure
❑ Postobstructive nephropathy

Each of the causes of polyuria produces a distinctive pattern to water restriction and exogenous ADH administration (*Table 34*):

❑ Cranial DI is usually partial, and therefore both ADH release and the urine osmolality may increase as the plasma osmolality rises, but submaximally. Exogenous ADH will lead to a rise in urine osmolality (and an equivalent fall in urine output) of more than 100% in complete central DI and 15–50% in partial central DI.

❑ Nephrogenic DI. A submaximal rise in urine osmolality in response to water restriction, with exogenous ADH producing little or no elevation in urine osmolality is seen. In complete nephrogenic DI, the urine osmolality is well below 300 mOsmol/l. There is a small (<45%) elevation in urine osmolality with partial nephrogenic DI.

❑ Primary polydipsia will be associated with a rise in urine osmolality, usually to above 500 mOsmol/l, and no response to exogenous ADH since endogenous release is intact.

If cranial DI has been diagnosed further investigations should include an MRI scan of the pituitary region. This may identify a hypothalamic or infiltrative tumour. There is frequently loss of the bright spot of the posterior pituitary gland.

OTHER METABOLIC DISEASE

There are a number of metabolic conditions that do not relate to disease of a single gland. These are covered in this section and include the following:

❑ Gastrointestinal neuroendocrine tumours.
❑ Electrolyte disturbances.
❑ Renal tubular abnormalities.
❑ Inherited endocrine syndromes.
❑ Dyslipidaemia.

GASTROINTESTINAL NEUROENDOCRINE TUMOURS

Neuroendocrine cells are found predominantly in the pancreas and gastrointestinal tract and are responsible for a number of well-documented syndromes (*Table 35*).

Insulinoma

Insulinomas arise from pancreatic acinar cells. The incidence of insulinoma is less than 4 cases per million per year and can arise in either sex with an age range of 18–61 years. Insulinomas are most frequently single and benign. In 15% of patients they are malignant and in 15% they are multiple. In 15% of cases, insulinoma is part of the Type 1 MEN syndrome. Clinical features include:

❑ Fasting hypoglycaemia.
❑ Neuroglycopaenic symptoms; confusion, visual and behaviour change.
❑ Occasionally autonomic symptoms; palpitations and tremor.
❑ Weight gain.
❑ Underlying neurological or psychiatric disorder (usually a misdiagnosis).

Investigations for insulinoma
The diagnosis of insulinoma in a patient with fasting hypoglycaemia is established by demonstrating

---

Table 34 Interpretation of urine osmolality results (mOsm/kg) in fluid deprivation tests

Diagnosis	After fluid deprivation	After desmopressin
Cranial diabetes insipidus	<300	>800
Nephrogenic diabetes insipidus	<300	<300
Primary polydipsia	>800	>800
Partial diabetes insipidus	300–800	<800

Table 35 Gastrointestinal neuroendocrine tumours

Condition	Hormone secreted
Insulinoma	Insulin
Glucagonoma	Glucagon
Carcinoid syndrome	Serotonin, tachykinins
Zollinger–Ellison syndrome	Gastrin
VIPoma	VIP
Somatostatinoma	Somatostatin
Cushing's syndrome	ACTH

inappropriately high serum insulin concentration during a spontaneous or induced episode of hypoglycaemia. If the plasma glucose is <2.5 mol/l and the plasma insulin is >5 mU/l, this indicates the presence of inappropriately excessive insulin. An elevated plasma insulin should be accompanied by an elevated plasma C-peptide unless the excess insulin has been given exogenously, e.g. following an overdose. A 72-hour fast may be required to induce hypoglycaemia in some patients. This is carried out as an inpatient. Plasma glucose, insulin, and C-peptide are measure 6 hourly during this test which can be terminated as soon as a plasma glucose <2.5 mmol/l is achieved.

After diagnosis, imaging techniques are then used to localize the tumour (**47a & b**).

The procedures available include MRI and CT scanning, arteriography, ultrasonography (transabdominal and endoscopic), and octreotide imaging. The choice of procedure depends upon local protocol and skills. Transabdominal ultrasonography is often the preferred initial test. All of these investigations can fail to identify the tumour. Although it is invasive, endoscopic ultrasonography appears to have the highest detection rate. Arterial calcium gluconate injection followed by hepatic venous sampling of insulin is sometimes used. A combination of investigations can localize the tumour site in >95% of patients prior to surgery.

When excessive insulin production is found, there are two rare differential diagnoses to consider:
❑ Familial persistent hyperinsulinaemic hypoglycaemia.
❑ Primary islet-cell hyperplasia (nesidioblastosis).

Glucagonoma

This is a tumour of the alpha cells of the pancreas. Glucagonomas are usually encapsulated, firm nodules, varying in size (2–25 cm) arising mostly in the tail of the pancreas.

Most pancreatic glucagonomas are malignant. They are rare and occur in either sex equally. Patients typically present in their fifth decade Rarely, glucagonoma may be associated with the Type 1 MEN syndrome. Clinical features of glucagonoma include:
❑ Necrolytic migratory erythema.
❑ Weight loss.
❑ Sore mouth.
❑ Diabetes mellitus (in 85%).
❑ Anaemia.
❑ Venous thrombosis (in 30%).

❑ Neuropsychiatric symptoms (dementia, ataxia, muscle weakness).
❑ Abdominal pain/diarrhoea/constipation.

The skin condition necrolytic migratory erythema characteristically begins as erythematous papules or plaques involving the face, perineum, and extremities These lesions enlarge and coalesce and leave bronze-coloured, indurated areas.

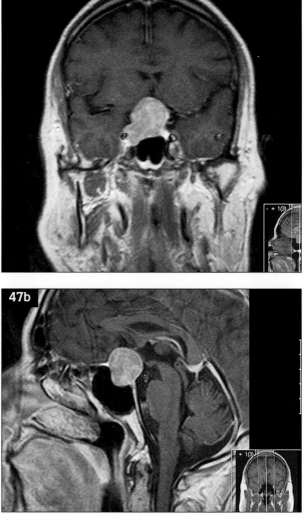

47 Gadolinium-enhanced MRI scans of the pituitary; (**a**) coronal section; (**b**) sagittal section. (Courtesy of Dr J. Thomas, St Bartholomew's Hospital, London.)

Investigations for glucagonoma

Glucagonomas are usually associated with markedly elevated serum concentrations of glucagon (>500 pg/ml, normal range <100 pg/ml). Occasionally, patients with the classic syndrome have a lower serum concentration (100–500 pg/ml). A full blood count reveals a normochromic, normocytic anaemia in more than 90% of cases.

Glucagonomas may produce multiple hormones including vasointestinal peptide (VIP), gastrin, serotonin, insulin, calcitonin, pancreatic polypeptide, and ACTH.

Clinical and/or laboratory abnormalities suggesting the presence of glucagonoma should be followed by attempts to localize the tumour. Abdominal contrast CT scanning is the initial imaging procedure of choice (85% sensitivity). Endoscopic ultrasound can detect smaller pancreatic tumours. Angiography is highly sensitive for islet cell tumours, given their hypervascularity. Somatostatin receptor scintigraphy using radiolabelled octreotide is very sensitive for islet cell tumours, including glucagonomas, but since glucagonomas are usually large by the time of diagnosis this is rarely required. Once the primary tumour and/or metastases have been localized, needle biopsy is used to confirm the diagnosis, via endoscopic ultrasound or CT.

Zollinger–Ellison syndrome (gastrinoma)

This condition is characterized by ulceration of the upper jejunum and hypersecretion of gastric acid due to a gastrinoma (a nonbeta-islet cell tumour of the gut or pancreas). This is a progressive and frequently life-threatening condition. Gastrin has been identified as the hormonal agent responsible for the syndrome. Other neuroendocrine peptides such as VIP and glucagon may also be cosecreted

This condition may be seen in up to 1% of patients with peptic ulcer disease Most patients are diagnosed between the ages of 20 and 50 years. It is slightly more common in men (male:female, 2:1). In 20% of patients, it is associated with Type 1 MEN syndrome.

Gastrinomas are derived from endodermal stem cells known as enteroendocrine cells. They can arise in the pancreas (30%) or small intestine (70%), usually the duodenum. Duodenal gastrinomas tend to be quite small and are often multiple. They have less malignant potential than pancreatic gastrinomas. Clinical features include:

❑ Peptic ulceration. Over 90% of patients with the Zollinger–Ellison syndrome develop peptic ulcers. The ulcers recur much more often than in patients with sporadic ulcer disease.
❑ Diarrhoea.
❑ Metastatic disease. This is evident at the time of diagnosis in one-third of patients.

The liver is the most common site of spread. Bony spread may occur later.

Investigations for gastrinoma

The fasting serum gastrin concentration is used for routine screening in patients with Type 1 MEN or recurrent severe peptic ulceration despite therapy. A serum gastrin >70 pmol/l raises the possibility of gastrinoma. A value greater than 475 pmol/l is virtually diagnostic of the disorder. However, most patients with the Zollinger–Ellison syndrome have serum gastrin concentrations between 70 and 475 pmol/l). This degree of hypergastrinaemia can also be present in patients with secondary hypergastrinaemia, due to achlorhydria as in pernicious anaemia or atrophic gastritis. False positives may also be seen in renal insufficiency, massive small bowel resection, gastric outlet obstruction, and in patients receiving potent antisecretory drugs.

A secretin stimulation test can differentiate patients with gastrinomas from those with the many other causes of hypergastrinaemia, and should be performed in every patient suspected to have the Zollinger–Ellison syndrome who has a nondiagnostic fasting serum gastrin concentration. Secretin stimulates the release of gastrin by gastrinoma cells and, therefore, most patients with these tumours have a dramatic rise in serum gastrin in response to a secretin infusion. The test is performed by administering 0.4 µg of secretin per kg body weight intravenously over 1 minute; a baseline serum gastrin is measured twice before the secretin is administered and at intervals 2, 5, 10, 15, and 20 minutes later. A rise in serum gastrin by 200 pg/ml (95 pmol/l) or more is considered a positive test, and is highly sensitive and specific for the presence of a gastrinoma.

Serum chromogranin A is a general marker for neuroendocrine tumours that is elevated in most patients with gastrinomas and may be used as a confirmatory test. A calcium infusion study is occasionally used in patients with clinical gastrinomas but a negative secretin test.

After diagnosis it is important to localize the site of the gastrinoma. The two tests most widely used are:
❏ Somatostatin receptor imaging (octreotide scanning). This is a highly sensitive test that can also demonstrate metastases.
❏ Endoscopic ultrasound. This is valuable in imaging small pancreatic endocrine tumours, and permits FNA for histological identification.

A combination of these two imaging procedures localizes more than 90% of tumours. Other techniques for localizing tumours include CT scanning, MRI, angiography, and arterial stimulation with venous sampling. Occasionally, localization can only be achieved at laparotomy by direct palpation or ultrasound imaging.

Carcinoid syndrome

Carcinoid tumours are the most common gastrointestinal neuroendocrine tumour. The age distribution ranges from the second to the ninth decade, with the peak incidence occurring between the ages of 50 and 70. Carcinoid tumours may arise anywhere in the gastrointestinal tract, in the bronchi, and occasionally elsewhere. The liver inactivates the bioactive products of carcinoid tumours. This may explain why patients who have gastrointestinal carcinoid tumours have the carcinoid syndrome only if they have hepatic metastases, resulting in the secretion of tumour products into the hepatic veins. As many as 40 secretory products have been identified in various carcinoid tumours. The most prominent of these are serotonin, histamine, tachykinins, kallikrein, and prostaglandins.

Eighty percent of patients with the carcinoid syndrome have small bowel carcinoids. Symptoms of the carcinoid syndrome only occur in 10% of patients. Gastric and bronchial carcinoids are associated with atypical carcinoid syndromes. In patients with intestinal carcinoid tumours, the carcinoid syndrome does not occur in the absence of liver metastases. Bronchial and other extraintestinal carcinoids, the bioactive products of which are not immediately cleared by the liver, can cause the syndrome in the absence of metastatic disease. The major symptoms are listed below:
❏ Cutaneous flushing. This occurrs in 85% of patients. The typical flush involves the face, neck, and upper chest and is associated with a mild burning sensation. Flushing can be provoked by eating, drinking, liver palpation, or stress. It may last for hours and be accompanied by severe hypotension (carcinoid crisis).
❏ Venous telangiectasia. Purplish vascular lesions occur late in the course of the carcinoid syndrome. These most often occur on the nose, upper lip, and malar areas.
❏ Diarrhoea. Secretory diarrhoea occurs in 80% of patients. Stools are typically watery and can be explosive and accompanied by abdominal pain.
❏ Bronchospasm. 15% have wheezing and dyspnoea.
❏ Cardiac valvular lesions. Carcinoid heart disease is characterized by deposits of fibrous tissue on the endocardium of valvular cusps, cardiac chambers and, occasionally, the pulmonary arteries or aorta. The valves and endocardium of the right side of the heart are most often affected.
❏ Rarer symptoms include glossitis, angular stomatitis, muscle wasting, mental confusion, and retroperitoneal fibrosis leading to ureteral obstruction or Peyronie's disease.

Investigations for carcinoid syndrome

The most useful initial diagnostic test for the carcinoid syndrome is to measure 24-hour urinary excretion of 5-HIAA, which is the end product of serotonin metabolism. This test has a sensitivity of 75% and specificity of up to 100%, but is affected by the consumption of tryptophan-rich food and several drugs (*Table 36*). The normal rate of 5-HIAA excretion is 10–42 μmol/day. Most patients with the carcinoid syndrome secrete >500 μmol/day. Measurement of urinary 5-HIAA excretion may not be useful in foregut carcinoids (bronchial, gastric).

Provocation of flushing using epinephrine or pentagastrin are useful in evaluating patients who describe flushing, but have normal or only marginally elevated biochemical markers. The pentagastrin provocation test is performed by administration of pentagastrin (0.06 mg/kg body weight) intravenously.

Table 36 Food and drugs to avoid when measuring urinary 5-HIAA

❏ Bananas	❏ Walnuts
❏ Avocado	❏ Salicylates
❏ Coffee	❏ Chlorpromazine
❏ Chocolate	❏ L-Dopa

To localize a carcinoid, CT scanning and pentetreotide (octreotide) imaging are used. Endoscopic MRI and angiography imaging are used in patients with tumours that have not been localized by other methods. Chest X-ray and CT scan can be used to localize bronchial carcinoid tumours. These tumours tend to be centrally located endobronchial lesions.

VIPoma

VIPomas are rare neuroendocrine tumours that secrete vasointestinal peptide (VIP). They are detected in 1 per 10 million population per year. The majority arise within the pancreas, although other VIP-secreting tumours have been reported. These include bronchogenic carcinoma, colon carcinoma, ganglioneuroblastoma, phaeochromocytoma, hepatoma, and adrenal tumours. Approximately 75% of VIPomas have metastasized by the time of diagnosis. VIPomas occur as part of the Type 1 MEN syndrome in 5%. VIPomas most commonly occur between 30 and 50 years, and in children aged 2 and 4 years. Most patients are symptomatic with watery diarrhoea, hypokalaemia, and hypochlorhydria. Other symptoms include flushing episodes, lethargy, nausea, vomiting, muscle weakness, and muscle cramps.

Investigations for VIPoma

VIPoma is diagnosed by the presence of an otherwise unexplained high volume secretory diarrhoea and a serum VIP concentration in excess of 75 pg/ml. Most pancreatic VIPomas are >3 cm in size at presentation and be identified by CT scanning. Octreotide scanning and endoscopic ultrasound are also used.

Somatostatinoma

These are rare neuroendocrine tumours of D-cell origin that contain and sometimes secrete excessive amounts of somatostatin. They usually arise within the pancreas gland and duodenum. Only about 10% of patients with somatostatinomas experience somatostatinoma syndrome. Patients present most commonly with abdominal pain and weight loss. Tumours localized within the pancreas sometimes cause the the somatostatinoma syndrome which has three components:
❏ Diabetes mellitus.
❏ Cholelithiasis.
❏ Diarrhoea with steatorrhoea.

Patients with duodenal somatostatinomas typically present with symptoms caused by local mass effects rather than the actions of the hormone; abdominal pain and jaundice are common presentations.

Investigations for somatostatinoma

If a somatostatinoma is suspected preoperatively on the basis of the classical triad of diabetes, gallstones, and steatorrhoea, or if an islet cell tumour mass is suspected, a fasting plasma somatostatin level should be measured. A concentration exceeding 160 pg/ml is suggestive of the diagnosis. Several imaging studies can be used to localize a suspected somatostatinoma: ultrasound, CT scan, MRI, and octreotide scanning.

ELECTROLYTE DISTURBANCES

Hyponatraemia

Hyponatraemia is a common metabolic abnormality recognized in both inpatients and outpatients. When considering the causes it is important to consider the clinical state of the patient and in particular the level of hydration, i.e. is the patient hypovolaemic (dehydrated), hypervolaemic (with signs of fluid excess, e.g. peripheral oedema, ascites) or euvolaemic (neither dehydrated nor fluid overloaded) (*Table 37*).

Table 37 Causes of hyponatraemia

In hypervolaemic patients:
❏ Excess intake of water (compulsive water drinking, excess intravenous dextrose)
❏ Increased reabsorption of water (cirrhosis, nephrotic syndrome, cardiac failure)
❏ Reduced renal excretion of water (SIADH)

In hypovolaemic patients:
❏ Renal loss of sodium (tubulointerstitial nephritis, acute polyuric recovery from renal tubular acidosis, relief of ureteric obstruction, analgesic nephropathy, mineralocorticoid deficiency)
❏ Nonrenal loss of sodium (fistulae, diarrhoea/vomiting, excessive sweating)

In euvolaemic patients:
❏ Glucocorticoid deficiency (Addison's disease/hypopituitarism/ discontinuation of steroid therapy)
❏ Fluid loss with adequate fluid replacement and inadequate electrolyte replacement (SIADH, corrected dehydration)

Clinical features include those of the underlying cause and features of fluid depletion (dehydration, hypotension, tachycardia) or fluid overload (peripheral and pulmonary oedema). Once the serum sodium drops below 115 nmol/l, neurological symptoms are likely. With a sodium concentration >125 mmol/l, symptoms of hyponatraemia are unlikely to occur. Common clinical features of hyponatraemia include:

❑ Confusion.
❑ Headache.
❑ Seizures.
❑ Coma.

Clinical inspection of the patient, coupled with a urinary sodium measurement helps differentiate between causes of hyponatraemia (*Table 38*).

Syndrome of inappropriate ADH (SIADH)
This condition is characterized by hyponatraemia occurring in the absence of oedema or volume depletion. The ADH secretion is inappropriate in the context of reduced serum osmolarity (a dilute serum). It is common in hospital inpatients and there are a large number of potential causes. The commonest causes are drug-related stimulation of ADH or ectopic secretion of ADH (*Table 39*).

Characteristic clinical and biochemical findings in SIADH include the following:

❑ Hyponatraemia.
❑ Reduced plasma osmolality (<270 mOsmol/l).
❑ Increased renal sodium loss (>20 mmol/l).

❑ No obvious fluid loss.
❑ Normal renal, adrenal, and thyroid function.

Baseline investigations should include a chest X-ray, full blood count, thyroid function, and a septic screen. Other investigations are usually not required since the condition is typically self-limiting and responsive to treatment of the underlying presenting condition. Further investigations should be directed at symptoms and potential causes.

RENAL TUBULAR ABNORMALITIES
Bartter's syndrome
This is a rare autosomal recessive abnormality that usually presents in early childhood. It is caused by a cotransporter abnormality in the ascending loop of Henle.

It leads to salt-wasting, and a hypokalaemic metabolic alkalosis. Symptoms include weakness, tetany, and seizures. Investigations reveal increased plasma renin activity and aldosterone plus raised urinary calcium.

Gitelman's syndrome
This is similar to Bartter's but can present at an older age. There is a loss of function of sodium transporters in the distal tubule, leading to hypokalaemic alkalosis, hypomagnesaemia, and hypocalciuria. Investigations reveal raised serum renin and aldosterone concentrations.

Table 38 Urinary sodium measurement in hyponatraemia

Hypovolaemia		Hypervolaemia		Euvolaemia	
Urine Na <20 mmol/l	Urine Na >20 mmol/l	Urine Na <20 mmol/l	Urine Na >20 mmol/l	Urine Na <20 mmol/l	Urine Na >20 mmol/l
Nonrenal sodium loss	Renal sodium loss	Compulsive water drinking	SIADH	Inadequate replacement of fluid loss	SIADH
	Mineralocorticoid deficiency	Congestive cardiac failure			Glucocorticoid deficiency
		Cirrhosis			
		Nephrotic syndrome			

Liddles's syndrome

This is a rare autosomal dominant condition caused by a defect in sodium channels of the distal nephron. It leads to hypokalaemic acidosis and hypertension. Investigations reveal suppressed renin and aldosterone.

INHERITED ENDOCRINE SYNDROMES

Type 1 MEN syndrome

This is an autosomal dominant condition with a prevalence of 1 in 10 000 of the UK population. It is characterized by disease of two or more endocrine glands as detailed below:

- ❏ Parathyroid hyperplasia/adenoma.
- ❏ Pancreatic endocrine tumours (gastrinoma, insulinoma, occasionally VIPoma, glucagonoma).
- ❏ Pituitary adenomas in 30% (prolactinoma, acromegaly, occasionally Cushing's, or nonfunctioning tumour).
- ❏ Others (foregut carcinoid, nodular adrenal hyperplasia, lipomas).

Type 2 MEN syndrome

There are two forms of this autosomal dominant condition (*Table 40*). Type 2b frequently presents as a sporadic new mutation. Medullary thyroid carcinoma is frequently the presenting feature. Development of phaeochromocytoma confirms the diagnosis. Mucosal neuromas are pathognomonic of MEN-2b. It is important to screen direct relatives of any patients with a MEN syndrome for the presence of the condition.

Medullary thyroid carcinoma

This can occur sporadically, in a dominantly inherited fashion or as part of a Type 2 MEN syndrome. The diagnosis may first be made on histology. The tumour is widespread with C-cell hyperplasia and stromal amyloid on histological analysis. Diarrhoea is present in one-third of patients. The patient occasionally presents with cushingoid features, since the tumour occasionally causes ectopic ACTH production. The diagnosis is suspected with elevated levels of basal calcitonin. It is confirmed by a pentagastrin test in which the calcitonin level rises at 2 minutes in response to 0.5 µg pentagastrin given intravenously.

DYSLIPIDAEMIA

Lipid abnormalities may occur as primary inherited states or secondary to other conditions. The more common primary dyslipidaemias are described here.

Table 39   Causes of SIADH

Chest disease:
- ❏ Pneumonia/empyema
- ❏ Asthma
- ❏ Positive pressure ventilation
- ❏ TB

CNS disease:
- ❏ Meningitis/encephalitis/abscess
- ❏ Head injury
- ❏ Subarachnoid haemorrhage
- ❏ Guillain–Barré

Drugs:
- ❏ Phenothiazines
- ❏ Carbamazepine
- ❏ Clofibrate
- ❏ Chloropramide
- ❏ Vincristine
- ❏ Cyclophosphamide

Malignancy:
- ❏ Small-cell lung carcinoma
- ❏ Leukaemia
- ❏ Mesothelioma
- ❏ Sarcoma
- ❏ Thymoma

Others:
- ❏ Hypothyroidism
- ❏ Glucocorticoid deficiency

Table 40   Features of Type 2 MEN syndrome

MEN-2a:
- ❏ Medullary thyroid carcinoma
- ❏ Phaeochromocytoma
- ❏ Parathyroid adenomas/hyperplasia

MEN-2b:
- ❏ Medullary thyroid carcinoma
- ❏ Phaeochromocytoma
- ❏ Mucosal ganglioneuromas (predominantly tongue, gastrointestinal tract, and conjunctivae)
- ❏ Marfanoid appearance
- ❏ Occasionally hyperparathyroidism (20%)

Familial hypercholesterolaemia (FH)

This is an autosomal dominant inherited condition that leads to an increase in LDL-cholesterol due to a mutation of LDL receptors. It affects one in 500 of the UK population and leads to premature coronary heart disease. More than half of heterozygotes die before the age of 60 years. Homozygotes usually present with symptoms before the age of 30 years. Total cholesterol levels are typically in excess of 8 mmol/l and may be double this in patients who are homozygous for the condition. Triglyceride levels tend to be normal. Clinical features include tendon xanthomata (fingers, hands, knees, Achilles), xanthelasma, and corneal arcus.

Polygenic hypercholesterolaemia

This is more common than FH and may be caused by a variety of mechanisms. Xanthelasma and xanthomata are not seen and the impact on the patient is less.

Familial combined hyperlipidaemia

This condition is a risk factor for cardiovascular disease and is the most common form of inherited hyperlipidaemia. It leads to an elevation of both LDL-cholesterol and triglycerides and there is typically a family history of premature cardiovascular disease in first-degree relatives.

Familial hypertriglyceridaemia

This an autosomal dominant condition characterized by elevated triglyceride and very low-density lipoprotein (VLDL) levels. LDL-cholesterol is frequently elevated. Clinical manifestations include red eruptive xanthomata and lipaemia retinalis.

Other dyslipidaemic conditions are listed in *Table 41*.

Investigation for dyslipidaemia

Dyslipidaemias may be triggered by other factors and conditions. In patients with raised LDL-cholesterol,

Table 41 Features of other dyslipidaemic conditions

Condition	Biochemical markers	Clinical features
Familial dysbetalipoproteinaemia	Elevated intermediate-density lipoprotein	Palmar striae xanthomata Tuberous xanthomata (on elbows, knees, and heels) Premature cardiovascular disease
Lipoprotein lipase defiency	Marked hypertriglyceridaemia and hyperchylomicronaemia Absence of lipoprotein lipase	Autosomal recessive Childhood presentation
Apo C-II deficiency	Marked hypertriglyceridaemia and hyperchylomicronaemia	Recurrent pancreatitis
Familial alphalipoprotein deficiency	Low HDL cholesterol and total cholesterol Raised triglycerides	Autosomal recessive Orange tonsils Hepatosplenomegaly Corneal opacities Neuropathies
Abetalipoproteinaemia	Low VLDL, LDL, and total cholesterol	Retinitis pigmentosa Ataxia Nystagmus Dysartria Neuropathies

lowered protective HDL-cholesterol, or raised triglycerides it is important to consider whether there are underlying causes or conditions and to address them before correcting the dyslipidaemia. There are well-established associations between atherosclerosis and plasma cholesterol, triglycerides, and LDL-cholesterol, with an inverse association with HDL-cholesterol. *Table 42* presents the causes of deranged lipids.

REPRODUCTIVE HORMONES
REPRODUCTIVE HORMONE EXCESS
Polycystic ovarian syndrome (PCOS)
This is a condition that leads to hyperandrogenism and menstrual irregularity in premenopausal women. It may be associated with multiple follicular ovarian cysts on ultrasound examination. It is the most common endocrine disorder affecting women. Some surveys have suggested that up to 1 in 5 women may be affected.

This condition is associated with increased frequency and amount of GnRH production from the hypothalamus. It is also associated with obesity and hyperinsulinaemia. This leads to an excess of LH and insulin which in turn stimulates the production of androgens from the ovaries and diminishes levels of SHBG. Clinical features include:

❏ Oligomenorrhoea or amenorrhoea (65%).
❏ Hirsuitism (60%).
❏ Obesity (40%).
❏ Subfertility (30%).
❏ Acne.
❏ Male pattern hair loss.

Hirsuitism tends to occur gradually (unlike virilizing tumours). Hairs are coarse and dark. They predominate in a male distribution pattern (face, chest, lower abdomen, thighs). A careful history and examination should focus on the rate of onset of symptoms, type of symptoms (especially virilizing features), and the presence of cushingoid features. Virilization should not be present (deepening of voice, broadening of shoulders, clitoromegaly).

Investigations for PCOS
Where hirsuitism is present, it is essential to exclude causes other than PCOS. These include ovarian and adrenal androgen-secreting tumours, late-onset CAH, and Cushing's syndrome. A testosterone level <5 nmol/l makes an androgen-secreting tumour unlikely. Women with PCOS usually have normal serum testosterone levels. LH concentration is raised,

---

Table 42 Causes of deranged lipids

Causes of elevated LDL- and total cholesterol	Causes of elevated triglycerides
❏ Diet (excessive saturated fats and calories)	❏ Diet
❏ Drugs (glucocorticoids, diuretics, cyclosporin)	❏ Obesity
❏ Hypothyroidism	❏ Alcohol
❏ Nephrotic syndrome	❏ Drugs (glucocorticoids, oestrogens)
❏ Chronic liver disease	❏ Hypothyroidism
❏ Pregnancy (from second trimester)	❏ Type 2 diabetes/insulin resistance
❏ Glycogen storage diseases	❏ Chronic renal failure
	❏ Pregnancy (from third trimester)
Causes of reduced HDL-cholesterol	❏ Lipodystrophies (rare)
❏ Obesity	❏ Peritoneal dialysis
❏ Smoking	
❏ Drugs (anabolic steroids)	
❏ Type 2 diabetes/insulin resistance	
❏ Chronic renal failure	

typically with an LH/FSH ration >1.5. SHBG is low in most women with PCOS, causing an elevation of circulating free testosterone. Serum PRL is frequently mildly elevated (up to 2000 mU/l). Transvaginal ultrasound examination (48) of the ovaries will show the presence of multiple (>8) follicular cysts in most women with PCOS, but the absence of cysts does not exclude the diagnosis. This investigation will also reveal most ovarian tumours. 17-hydroxyprogesterone levels are raised in late-onset CAH, but not in PCOS. Dihydroepiandrostenedione (DHEA) sulphate and androstenedione are androgens that may be mildly elevated in PCOS. DHEA sulphate is an adrenal androgen. Significantly elevated levels (>20 μmol/l) suggests an adrenal tumour.

Trans-vaginal ultrasound may demonstrate typical multifollicular cystic appearance of PCOS. MRI scanning of ovaries and adrenal glands detects most virilizing tumours. Selective venous sampling of adrenal and ovarian veins can be used to detect elevated testosterone levels. Screening tests for Cushing's syndrome can be performed if there is a clinical suspicion. Women with PCOS have an increased risk of Type 2 diabetes and cardiovascular disease. They should be screened for diabetes and dyslipidaemia.

Androgen-secreting tumours

These tumours usually arise in the ovary or adrenal gland. They frequently occur in young women (<50 years). They may be benign or malignant. Malignancy is associated with size. Ovarian tumours are usually sex cord stromal cell tumours and less commonly teratomas and gonadoblastomas. Adrenal tumours may copresent with features of Cushing's syndrome. Common clinical features include:

❏ Rapid onset of symptoms.
❏ Hyperandrogenism (hirsuitism, menstrual irregularity, and subfertility).
❏ Virilization.
❏ Abdominal pain, mass, and ascites.

FEMALE REPRODUCTIVE HORMONE DEFICIENCIES
Premature ovarian failure (POF) and the menopause

Premature ovarian failure (POF) is defined by amenorrhoea, oestrogen deficiency, and elevated gonadotrophins (particularly FSH) in women aged <40 years as a result of ovarian failure. Premature ovarian failure occurs in 1% of women. The menopause is the permanent cessation of menstruation for

a period of 12 months. This typically occurs between the ages of 45 and 55 years. *Table 43* presents the causes of POF.

Clinical features of POF and menopause include:
❏ Amenorrhoea.
❏ Symptoms of oestrogen deficiency:
  ❏ Night sweats.
  ❏ Hot flushes.
  ❏ Mood changes.
  ❏ Fatigue.
  ❏ Dyspareunia.

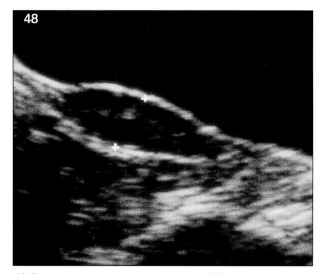

48 Ovarian ultrasound in a patient with PCOS, showing a 'necklace' of cysts around the periphery of the ovary. (Courtesy of Manson Publishing: *Paediatrics and Child Health*, 2007.)

Table 43 Causes of premature ovarian failure

❏ Turner's syndrome
❏ Fragile X syndrome
❏ Autoimmune disease
❏ Chemotherapy
❏ Following radiotherapy
❏ Gene mutations
❏ Chromosomal mutations
❏ Congenital adrenal hyperplasia
❏ Viral infections (mumps, human immunodeficiency virus)
❏ Surgical oophorectomy

Table 44 Clinical investigations in premature ovarian failure

Test	Result
Serum gonadotrophins	Elevated LH, higher FSH
Serum oestradiol	Low
Karyotype from blood film or buccal smear	Partial or complete absence of X chromosome in Turner's Y chromosome present in testicular feminization
Pelvic ultrasound	To demonstrate normal ovarian tissue (ovarian streaks may be seen in Turner's)
Thyroid and adrenal autoantibodies	Often positive; indicates risk of other glandular failure
Other tests as indicated	Turner's and autoimmune patients may require regular screening for associated complications and conditions

❏ Symptoms relating to other conditions (previous therapies, autoimmune disease).
❏ Increased risk of osteoporosis.

Autoimmune ovarian failure
This may be associated with Type 1 or Type 2 autoimmune polyglandular syndrome, or with other single organ autoimmune conditions (Addison's disease, thyroid disease, Type 1 diabetes, and myasthenia gravis).

Turner's syndrome
This condition is characterized by the absence of one X chromosome. It may be partial or total. It affects 1 in 2500 women. Clinical features include:
❏ Short stature.
❏ Failure of ovarian development.
❏ Premature ovarian failure.
❏ Webbed neck.
❏ Micrognathia.
❏ Cubitus valgus.
❏ Widely spaced nipples.
❏ Cognitive/social impairment but normal intelligence.

Women with Turner's syndrome are at increased risk of left sided congenital heart defects, aortic coarctation, hypothyroidism, diabetes, osteoporosis, and renal abnormalities.

Investigations for POF
Investigations used in the diagnosis of POF are presented in *Table 44*. When evaluating women with

Table 45 Causes of amenorrhoea not due to ovarian failure

❏ Pregnancy
❏ Kallman's syndrome
❏ Polycystic ovarian syndrome
❏ Congenital absence of uterus
❏ Uterine disease
❏ Hypopituitarism
❏ Hyperprolactinaemia
❏ Hypothyroidism
❏ Weight loss
❏ Anorexia
❏ Excessive exercise
❏ Physical illness
❏ Hypothalamic disease

POF it is important to remember that a wide range of conditions may present with amenorrhoea. Oestrogen deficiency may or may not be present; *Table 45* lists conditions that should be considered in the differential diagnoses.

MALE HYPOGONADISM

This is a condition where there is failure to produce adequate testosterone or spermatozoa. Male hypogonadism is due to inadequate production of testosterone. It can be either primary hypogonadism (a testicular cause) or secondary to pituitary or hypothalamic disease. Causes of primary hypogonadism are presented in *Table 46*.

Klinefelter's syndrome (**49a & b**) is a condition that affects 1 in 500 men and is characterized by additional X chromosomal material, typically XXY. It results in the following clinical features:
- ❑ Small testes.
- ❑ Gynaecomastia.
- ❑ Microspadia.
- ❑ Reduced intelligence quotient (40%).

Causes of secondary hypogonadism are presented in *Table 47*.

Kallman's syndrome

This is a condition affecting 1 in 10 000 people characterized by failure of GnRH secretion. It is more common in men than women (4:1). Most patients (75%) have anosmia. Some have delayed puberty. Occasionally it is seen in association with cleft pale, sensorineural deafness, ataxia, or renal abnormalities. It is genetically inherited (recessive, dominant, or X-linked).

Clinical features of hypogonadism

A careful history should be taken with a focus on previous developmental difficulties, delayed puberty, trauma, infection, and medical and drug history. A sexual history (erectile function, intercourse, fertility) should also be ascertained. Physical examination should include inspection of testes and penis size and appearance, body and pubic hair distribution, gynaecomastia, muscle mass, and fat distribution.

Table 46 Causes of primary male hypogonadism

- ❑ Klinefelter's syndrome (XXY or XY/XXY)
- ❑ Other chromosomal disorders:
  XX/XO (mixed gonadal dysgenesis)
  XX (with partial translocation of Y chromosome into an X)
  XYY (usually tall)
  XY Noonan's syndrome (male with features of Turner's syndrome)
- ❑ Bilateral cryptorchidism (undescended testes)
- ❑ Orchitis (postpubertal mumps or human immunodeficiency virus infection, autoimmune disease)
- ❑ Chemotherapy (affects 50%; pretreatment sperm donation should be offered if future fertility required)
- ❑ Local radiotherapy
- ❑ Varicocoele
- ❑ Trauma (local trauma, testicular torsion, or surgery)
- ❑ Chronic renal failure
- ❑ Chronic liver disease
- ❑ Haemachromatosis
- ❑ Alcohol
- ❑ Drug-induced (rare)

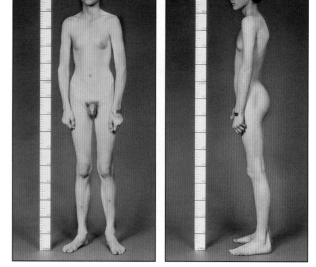

49 a, b Clinical features of Klinefelter's syndrome. (Courtesy of Manson Publishing: *Paediatrics and Child Health*, 2007.)

This will enable the detection of local disease, feminization or other underlying disease. Typical findings in the adult are:

❏ Small (<15 ml) soft testes.
❏ Gynaecomastia.
❏ Reduced body hair.
❏ Osteoporosis.

Where testosterone is reduced prior to puberty, the above features are found but in addition there is reduced penis size (<5 cm), high-pitched voice, central fat distribution, increased arm span and upper body length compared with height, and reduced bone age on X-ray examination.

Investigations for hypogonadism

Serum testosterone is low for all causes of hypogonadism. It is best checked at 9 am when peak levels occur. Since much of the hormone is bound to SHBG, this should also be measured and free testosterone measured when SHBG is low. In primary hypogonadism, LH and FSH levels are elevated. These are normal or low in secondary hypogonadism. In children, where it is necessary to differentiate primary from secondary hypogonadism, beta-human chorionic gonadotrophin (beta-HCG) can be given intramuscularly on two occasions 48 hours apart to assess testosterone response.

Table 47 Causes of secondary male hypogonadism

❏ Kallmann's syndrome
❏ Idiopathic hypogonadotrophic hypogonadism
❏ Excessive exercise
❏ Weight loss
❏ Systemic illness (acute or chronic)
❏ Pituitary or hypothalamic tumours
❏ Pituitary or hypothalamic surgery/trauma
❏ Radiotherapy
❏ Sarcoidosis
❏ Haemachromatosis
❏ Congenital syndromes (Prader–Willi, Lawrence–Moon–Biedl)
❏ Congenital adrenal hyperplasia

DIABETES

THE PREVENTION OF TYPE 1 DIABETES

THE PREVENTION OF TYPE 2 DIABETES

IDENTIFYING PEOPLE WITH TYPE 2 DIABETES

MANAGING THE ACUTE COMPLICATIONS OF DIABETES

GENERAL DIABETES MANAGEMENT AND LIFESTYLE

PHARMACOLOGICAL TREATMENT IN TYPE 1 DIABETES

PHARMACOLOGICAL TREATMENT IN TYPE 2 DIABETES

MANAGING THE CHRONIC COMPLICATIONS OF DIABETES

MANAGING DIABETES IN PREGNANCY

ENDOCRINOLOGY

MANAGING THYROID DISEASE

MANAGING PARATHYROID DISEASE

MANAGING ADRENAL DISEASE

MANAGING PITUITARY DISEASE

MANAGING METABOLIC DISEASE

MANAGING REPRODUCTIVE DISEASE

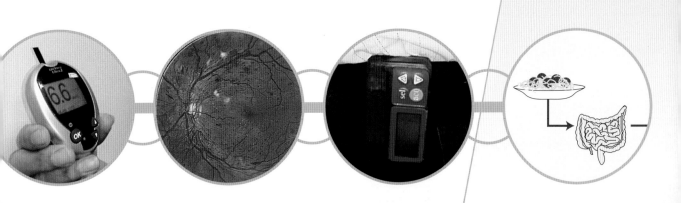

DIABETES

THE PREVENTION OF TYPE 1 DIABETES

The autoimmune process in Type 1 diabetes begins years before β-cells are destroyed. Measuring HLA susceptibility markers and autoantibody tests allows those at high risk of developing the disease to be identified. At present there is no reliable method of preventing its development. Studies in small groups of children have shown that aggressive insulin therapy in those likely to develop Type 1 diabetes may delay the development of the condition as a result of reduced β-cell activity.

Cyclosporin has been shown to induce remission for one year in 50% of patients with Type 1 diabetes of short duration. However, the effect only lasts for the duration of therapy and the nephrotoxicity of the drug has halted further trials. Nicotinamide has also been shown to delay the progression to Type 1 diabetes in susceptible individuals, probably through its action on deoxyribonucleic acid (DNA) synthesis and increasing β-cell regeneration. Although there is great interest in the area of Type 1 diabetes prevention, there are still no definitive positive results from intervention studies and trials.

THE PREVENTION OF TYPE 2 DIABETES

The global epidemic of Type 2 diabetes, driven by changes in diet and physical inactivity, is potentially preventable through the institution of appropriate public health measures. These can be targeted at small groups of high-risk individuals or at whole communities. Studies have now shown that measures aimed at altering lifestyle can prevent the progression of glucose intolerance to full blown Type 2 diabetes. In the Finnish Diabetes Prevention Study, an individualized programme combining weight reduction, a healthy diet, and increased physical exercise reduced the risk by nearly 60%. Exercise has also been shown to prevent Type 2 diabetes independently in those who are overweight or who have impaired glucose tolerance.

It is possible to identify individuals at higher risk of developing diabetes since there are a number of predictive risk factors (*Table 48*). Preventative advice for those at risk of Type 2 diabetes should include the following:

❏ Recommendation of a healthy diet which is high in fibre and low in saturated fat.
❏ Regular aerobic exercise.
❏ Avoiding cigarette smoking.
❏ Avoiding obesity.

Table 48 Risk factors for developing Type 2 diabetes

Nonmodifiable	Potentially modifiable
Ethnicity – high-risk ethnic group, e.g. Pima Indian, South Pacific Islands, Australian Aboriginee, Arab peninsula or South Asia	Obesity (glucose intolerance and insulin resistance)
Family history – a first degree relative with Type 2 diabetes	Sedentary lifestyle
Age – older than 40 years (risk increases inexorably with age)	Endocrine disease, e.g. acromegaly, Cushing's syndrome, and phaeochromocytoma
Previous gestational diabetes	High-dose glucocorticoid treatment
Small birth weight	Cigarette smoking

IDENTIFYING PEOPLE WITH TYPE 2 DIABETES

There is currently no national screening programme for identifying Type 2 diabetes in the UK. However, there is increased public awareness of the condition and there are plans outlined in the government's National Service Framework for Diabetes to identify people who do not know that they have the condition. Many more people are now being screened for the presence of diabetes. It seems sensible to have a targeted screening approach. The following high-risk groups are likely to benefit from such a programme:

❏ Those with a first-degree relative with diabetes.
❏ The obese (>20% above ideal bodyweight).
❏ Those with previous impaired glucose tolerance (IGT) and impaired fasting glucose (IFG).
❏ Women with a history of gestational diabetes.
❏ Women who have delivered an overweight baby (>4 kg).
❏ Older members (>60 years) of high-risk ethnic groups, i.e. Indo-Asian and Afro-Caribbean.
❏ Those with circulatory disease (ischaemic heart disease, cerebrovascular, or peripheral vascular disease).
❏ Those with organ-specific autoimmune disease, e.g. primary hypothyroidism.
❏ Those with peripheral skin ulceration.
❏ Those suffering from severe or recurrent sepsis.

Screening should probably take the form of a fasting plasma glucose in the first instance with subsequent screening every 3 years.

MANAGING THE ACUTE COMPLICATIONS OF DIABETES

HYPOGLYCAEMIA

Mild hypoglycaemia

The management of hypoglycaemia depends upon its duration, severity, and the location in which it takes place. The patient can usually correct mild hypoglycaemia, provided that warning symptoms are recognized and that carbohydrate is available. If the patient is hospitalized and unable to obtain carbohydrate easily, it is important that medical and nursing staff are able to recognize hypoglycaemia and supply carbohydrate quickly. The choice of carbohydrate relates to the speed of its absorption. Simple sugars in the form of dextrose tablets, chocolate, Hypostop, or Lucozade are easy and effective. However, more complex carbohydrate such as digestive biscuits or a sandwich may be as effective.

It is not uncommon for friends or relatives to recognize hypoglycaemia before the sufferer, particularly when warning symptoms are lost. A change in behaviour may be observed and some become uncooperative during an attack. The sufferer should be encouraged to take a quick-acting sugary drink. Quick-acting sugars will often be effective for less than half an hour and secondary consumption of more complex carbohydrate-containing food, such as a sandwich, will give a more sustained effect.

Severe hypoglycaemia

Administering fluids or food to unresponsive subjects risks aspiration. Hypostop is a glucose gel that can be squirted into the buccal cavity where it is safely absorbed. It can be a useful preparation in severe hypoglycaemia occurring outside of a hospital setting. Some patients, particularly those with recurrent hypoglycaemia or during pregnancy, can be prescribed an intramuscular preparation of glucagon in case of severe hypoglycaemia. It is supplied as a powder and fluid that are combined prior to administration. In the community setting it can be given intramuscularly or subcutaneously and is effective within 10 minutes. In the hospital setting it should be given intravenously. It is less effective in prolonged hypoglycaemia and in malnourished patients, alcohol abusers, and those with liver, pituitary, or adrenal gland failure.

The preferred treatment for severe hypoglycaemia is intravenous dextrose, given as a dose of 25–50 ml of 50% dextrose concentration. This should be effective within 5 minutes. Following resolution of hypoglycaemia, patients may complain of headache or nausea. Once alert, the patient should be encouraged to ingest carbohydrate.

Persistent hypoglycaemia, particularly in the context of a large insulin or sulphonylurea overdose, will require a continuous infusion of 10% dextrose, occasionally accompanied by further boluses of 50% dextrose. Hourly capillary blood glucose measurements should be taken until the patient is fully recovered and no further infusions are required.

If consciousness does not return quickly, differential diagnoses should be considered. These include cerebral oedema secondary to severe hypoglycaemia, a postictal state, a cerebrovascular event, head injury, and overdose. Cerebral oedema is seen on CT scanning. Management is supportive with artificial ventilation. High-dose dexamethasone, intravenous mannitol, and intermittent positive-pressure ventilation (IPPV) are sometimes used.

acute phase. An alternative is an intravenous sliding scale system of insulin administration according to local protocols. Controversy persists over the continuing use of insulin following hospital discharge. DIGAMI suggested improved outcomes for hyperglycaemic patients receiving insulin infusion during the phase immediately following an MI and continuing subcutaneous insulin for up to 2 years. Separate studies have confirmed the benefit of correcting hyperglycaemia in the acute phase. DIGAMI 2, United Kingdom Prospective Diabetes Study (UKPDS), and other studies have not shown any benefit for routinely continuing insulin therapy beyond the acute phase.

Metformin should be withdrawn in patients with acute coronary disease because of the increased risk of lactic acidosis. Sulphonylureas should probably be stopped immediately post MI while insulin is infused. Thiazolidinedione drugs should be stopped in view of the increased risk of cardiac failure.

After insulin is discontinued (at 48–72 hours) diabetic patients can return to their previous sulphonylurea therapy. Treatment-naïve patients need to be assessed for individual requirements according to their blood glucose. Angioplasty and coronary artery bypass grafting appear less effective in patients with Type 2 diabetes. Graft survival and patient survival rates are lower. This may be because atheromatous disease is more diffuse and distal. The introduction of newer techniques for revascularization, such as stenting, need further evaluation but may be beneficial in diabetes. However, patients should not be denied revascularization because of diabetes, particularly since it is equally effective for symptom relief.

PERIOPERATIVE MANAGEMENT

Managing insulin-treated patients perioperatively

Diabetic patients undergoing surgery should be managed according to a simple local protocol that is adhered to by all medical and nursing staff. Nonoperative complications are usually due to a failure to understand or follow agreed pathways.

It is advisable for diabetic patients to be operated upon first on a morning list. This minimizes the effects of starvation and ensures that ample medical and support staff are available during the postoperative period. Normal diet and insulin doses are taken the day prior to surgery. For those on insulin undergoing minor surgery, the patient should be operated on first thing in the morning with no breakfast and having received half their normal prebreakfast dose of insulin. Additional short-acting insulin may be required prior to lunch, taking into account the patient's usual insulin requirements and prevailing blood glucose levels. If the patient is on an afternoon list, a light breakfast should be given with half the usual dose of morning short-acting insulin.

All patients undergoing major surgery require insulin during surgery, and should receive intravenous insulin, glucose, and potassium. This should be started first thing in the morning, or at midday if the operation is planned for the afternoon. The traditional method for administering intravenous glucose, insulin, and potassium (GIK) has been the Alberti regime. This consists of 500 ml of 10% glucose into which is added 10–15 units of soluble quick-acting insulin and 10 mmol of potassium. This is usually infused at 100 ml/hour. This technique of combining insulin and dextrose reduces the risk of deranged blood glucose occurring due to insulin or dextrose being stopped. Its disadvantage is the lack of flexibility if that particular regime does not fit with individual metabolic requirements. With the advent of reliable syringe pumps, a sliding scale of insulin is now frequently used. With this, the infusion of dextrose and potassium is maintained with the separate introduction of insulin through a connecting tube that joins the dextrose and potassium infusion. This allows more easily for the adjustment of insulin doses according to a locally agreed regime.

Blood glucose levels need to be monitored half to one-hourly during surgery using a bedside blood glucose monitor. Target blood glucose levels should be 6–10 mmol/l. Serum potassium should be measured at least 2 hourly and levels of 4–5 mmol/l should be targeted.

Managing insulin-treated patients postoperatively

The hormonal responses to surgery can persist for several days. Postoperative glucose control is best achieved with a combination of an insulin sliding scale and a glucose and potassium infusion. Care should be taken to avoid hyponatraemia and to ensure appropriate levels of hydration. Once a patient is eating and drinking, they should be transferred back to their usual insulin regime. This should occur at mealtime, ideally breakfast, or when the patient usually administers a combination of short and intermediate-acting insulin. The insulin infusion should continue for 1–2 hours after the first subcutaneous injection.

Managing diet or tablet-controlled patients

All patients with diabetes who are undergoing major surgery should be managed as for insulin-treated patients. For those patients undergoing minor surgery, oral hypoglycaemic drugs should be omitted on the morning of surgery and a GIK infusion only started if there is significant hyperglycaemia. It is essential that blood glucose levels are monitored frequently, particularly if the operation is lengthy.

Tablets should be restarted after surgery. Patients with stable, well-controlled diabetes may be able to undergo minor surgery on the same day provided they are expected to be eating by lunch time after surgery. All patients require a preoperative assessment that includes an assessment of their self-management abilities and whether there is support at home on the day of surgery.

CASE 1

A 24-year-old girl presents to the Accident & Emergency Department unwell. She is vomiting and drifting in and out of unconsciousness. She is not able to give a good history but her boyfriend says that she has been feeling unwell for several weeks and has been losing weight. On examination she is dyspnoeic (respiratory rate = 32). She is tachycardic (pulse rate = 118 bpm) and hypotensive (blood pressure = 80/50 mmHg). Her abdomen is tense. Her routine blood test results are shown:

Results (normal range)
Sodium 135 mmol/l (135–146)
Potassium 7.3 mmol/l (3.6–5.0)
Urea 13.3 mmol/l (3.2–7.1)
Creatinine 135µmol/l (71–110)

1 What urgent investigation is required?
2 What is the likely diagnosis?
3 What immediate management steps are required?

CASE 2

A 71-year-old man is admitted to hospital having been unwell for 1 week. On arrival to the Medical Admissions Department he is very breathless. His wife says that during the course of the day he has become increasingly confused and sleepy. He now has a Glasgow Coma Score (GCS) of 4. On examination he is very dehydrated (dry mucous membranes, sunken eyes, and loss of skin turgor). Other abnormalities found on examination are that he is febrile (temperature 38.9°C), he has a tachycardia (pulse rate = 112 bpm) and loud harsh crepitations at both lung bases. Investigation results reveal a very high plasma glucose (61 mmol/l [3.6–6.1]) and a raised urea (33 mmol/l [3.2–7.1]).

1 i.   What is wrong with this patient?
  ii. How dehydrated is he?
  iii. How quickly should his fluid loss be replaced?
2 What investigations does he require?

Answers to Cases 1 & 2 on page 157.

GENERAL DIABETES MANAGEMENT AND LIFESTYLE

THE ASSESSMENT AND MANAGEMENT OF A NEW PATIENT WITH DIABETES

The assessment and management of a new patient with diabetes should follow the management plan outlined in *Table 49*.

Establishing the diagnosis

A plasma glucose measurement is the important investigation in establishing the diagnosis of diabetes. Diagnostic criteria are outlined earlier. Ideally, the sample should be collected into a tube containing fluoride oxalate and then measured in a clinical laboratory setting using a specific glucose assay. Capillary glucose measurements collected by fingerprick testing are convenient but need to be confirmed with a plasma sample. Glycosuria discovered on urine testing is not sufficient for a diagnosis. A glycosylated haemoglobin (HbA1c) or fructosamine are good indicators of long-term glucose control but are not sensitive enough for diagnostic purposes except in very high-risk groups.

It should be remembered that patients who are acutely unwell may have a transient elevation of plasma glucose that settles rapidly. However, this does tend to suggest a propensity to the development of diabetes at a later stage. Elevation of plasma glucose in a sick patient should usually be managed with insulin. Even if glucose concentration returns quickly to normal, a plasma glucose should be re-checked within 6 weeks. Whether a new patient presents with symptoms or acutely unwell, a diagnosis can usually be suspected quickly by urine dipstick testing or a capillary blood glucose measurement. Confirmation should be with a laboratory plasma glucose concentration that exceeds 11 mmol/l.

Diabetes is a chronic disease that may present acutely. If a patient with a new diagnosis of diabetes is severely ill, then the patient is likely to require urgent hospital admission. This is irrespective of blood glucose concentration. History, examination, and early investigations may help to clarify the severity of the acute presentation. Appropriate urgent management should be initiated.

History, examination, and investigations

A full medical history should be taken from the patient. This should include:
❑ Symptoms of hyperglycaemia (thirst, polyuria, fatigue, weight loss, visual disturbance).
❑ Symptoms relating to diabetic complications (sensory loss, ulceration, urinary tract infection, balanitis, candidiasis, impotence, angina, claudication).
❑ Symptoms of underlying endocrine disease.
❑ Past medical history (associated diabetic conditions and complications).
❑ Drug history (diuretic and steroid use).
❑ Family history (diabetes and cardiac disease).
❑ Social circumstances.
❑ Lifestyle (smoking, diet, exercise, alcohol history).

It is important to assess for any acute metabolic disturbanc. A thorough physical examination of cardiovascular, abdominal, respiratory, and neurological systems may reveal underlying disease or associated complications. As part of a routine assessment examination, the following essential observations should be made:
❑ Height.
❑ Weight (with calculation of body mass index [BMI] +/−; waist:hip circumference ratio).
❑ Foot examination (skin integrity, foot deformities, pulses, sensation).
❑ Eye examination (visual acuity, ophthalmic examination through dilated pupils).

Table 49 Management plan for a new diabetic patient

❑ Establish the diagnosis.
❑ Assess the severity of illness +/- urgent treatment
❑ History
❑ Examination
❑ Investigations
❑ Provide advice and reassurance
❑ Facilitate early education
❑ Initiate nonurgent treatment
❑ Make appropriate referrals
❑ Develop an individualized management plan
❑ Long-term follow-up

Table 50 Initial management plan for patients with newly diagnosed diabetes

- ❑ Initially provide basic, simple information
- ❑ Be positive about the benefits of care; address and allay any fears or anxieties
- ❑ Include immediate family and friends in discussions about the condition, its significance, and management
- ❑ Give a simple explanation of what diabetes is. The patient should be told about the effects that it would have upon them, what their care plan will look like, and how they will be involved
- ❑ Highlight adverse features of their current lifestyles and how these should be addressed, including smoking, diet, exercise, and foot care
- ❑ Advise patients of the need to notify the DVLA that they have diabetes and to carry a card indicating that they have diabetes and the treatment that they are on
- ❑ If appropriate, give information about symptoms of hypoglycaemia and advise the patient to carry glucose tablets or an equivalent quick-acting sugary substance
- ❑ Inform those commencing treatment that they can pick up and sign a FP92A (UK free prescription) form from a pharmacist. This is sent to the Health Authority who issues an exemption certificate
- ❑ Consider pneumococcal and influenza vaccination unless this is contraindicated

Table 51 Key points for diabetes education

- ❑ Information about the nature of diabetes
- ❑ Information about how diabetes will affect health and lifestyle
- ❑ A diabetes care plan
- ❑ An introduction to members of the diabetes team
- ❑ Exercise and healthy living
- ❑ Dietary management
- ❑ Weight control
- ❑ Care of feet
- ❑ Coping strategies
- ❑ Illness
- ❑ Capillary blood testing
- ❑ Issues around driving
- ❑ Insurance
- ❑ Travel
- ❑ Medication – how it works, why it is used, and potential side-effects
- ❑ Starting on insulin
- ❑ Complications of diabetes

There are a few essential baseline tests that should be carried out in someone with a suspected new diagnosis of Type 2 diabetes:
- ❑ Urine dipstick analysis for the presence of glucose, protein, and ketones.
- ❑ Blood chemistry: urea and electrolytes, liver function, thyroid function, and lipid profile.
- ❑ Full blood count.

A coeliac antibody screen is recommended in children. Specific autoantibodies or C-peptide measurements can be taken where there is doubt as to the nature of the condition (i.e. whether it is Type 1 or Type 2 diabetes).

Table 50 presents the advice that should be given to newly diagnosed diabetic patients.

Facilitating diabetes education

Education is a key component of the management of diabetes. A diabetes education programme should include some key topics (*Table 51*). One of the challenges of diabetes care is to ensure that education is ongoing. There is good evidence that the benefits of diabetes education are lost unless there is reinforcement. Those that provide diabetes care need to ensure that information is both reinforced and updated continuously. This may be achieved through one to one opportunistic exchanges with the nurse, doctor, dietician, or podiatrist. However, it is best provided through a continuous programme of individual or group education.

Patients should be central to their own care since self-management is essential.

Dietary advice should be provided from the onset of the diagnosis of diabetes. It should be provided by appropriately trained professionals and should be sensitive to personal needs and culture as well as being relevant to any comorbid conditions and diabetic complications. Efforts should be made to optimize food choices and to advise appropriate insulin doses for different quantities of each food. There is controversy as to whether 'carbohydrate counting' or 'healthy lifestyle' should be the focus of dietary advice for people with Type 1 diabetes. However, these ideas need not be mutually exclusive. The differing glycaemic effects of foods need to be understood as well as the effects of different insulin preparations to treat them. Healthy eating with plenty of low glycaemic index foods, fruit, vegetables, and low fat options can help to reduce vascular risk. Nevertheless, information should still be provided about the effect of high glycaemic index foods and alcohol.

The DAFNE education programme is one that teaches people how to adjust their insulin doses to fit with their own lifestyle. Originally developed in Germany, research has been carried out in a number of UK centres to investigate the effects of the DAFNE approach. Its success has led to locally modified versions of DAFNE being introduced in many centres. It is likely that more courses will be developed to educate patients with Type 1 diabetes about the effects of lifestyle and insulin therapy on glucose control.

Physical activity should be encouraged and information provided on how to increase physical activity with insulin and dietary changes that may be required.

Nonsmokers should be advised not to start smoking and smokers offered advice on smoking cessation and the services that are available. This should be re-inforced at annual visits. Insulin therapy should usually be started as an outpatient. The patient should meet early with a trained health care professional, usually a diabetes nurse specialist. This individual should continue providing support where possible.

At these initial meetings, a full programme of education is not appropriate. The diagnosis has usually come as a shock and the need for injection therapy may be difficult for some to cope with. It is important to include immediate family in discussions since it may be important for those close to the patient to have an understanding of the condition, its impact, management, and consequences. The initial consultation should include:

❑ A demonstration of an insulin delivery system (frequently pen +/- cartridges) and injection technique.
❑ Initiation of insulin therapy (the first dose).
❑ Response to specific questions and concerns.
❑ Advice about recognition and treatment of hypoglycaemia.
❑ Advice on driving (informing Driver and Vehicle Licensing Authority [DVLA]).

❑ Advice regarding return to work and whether work is appropriate.
❑ Simple dietary advice (i.e. regular meal consumption and avoidance of excessive sugary drinks/sweets).
❑ A contact number for advice/help.
❑ Advice to pick up a free prescription form from the pharmacist (FP92A).
❑ Providing an identification card with diagnosis and treatment details to be carried at all times.

There should initially be a weekly review with the nurse specialist, an early medical assessment, institution of capillary blood glucose monitoring, and full dietary instruction.

Nonurgent treatment

Once it has been established that a patient is well, it is important to establish whether immediate insulin treatment is required. Clues to this, mentioned previously, are young age, slim build, and the presence of severe symptoms including weight loss and ketonuria. Overweight middle-aged or elderly Type 2 patients are likely to be initial candidates for aggressive dietary management. However, there is no guarantee that this is always correct. Caution is required and where there is doubt, frequent early follow-up is recommended. Drug therapy is discussed in much more detail later in this chapter.

In the UK, there has been an increasing trend for diabetes management to take place in primary care. Provided that there is an adequate understanding and knowledge of diabetes there is evidence that this condition can be well managed away from the specialist hospital setting. Practitioners should be aware of situations where a referral to hospital care is recommended (*Table 52*).

Every newly diagnosed patient with Type 2 diabetes requires a basic level of care but this requires personal modification depending upon individual characteristics, attitudes, and choice of treatment. It is essential that the patient is placed at the centre of their own care. Self-management is a vital aspect of good diabetes care and the patient should play the fullest possible role.

In the early stages, management of diabetes is aimed at abolishing symptoms of the condition and then achieving optimal blood glucose control, avoiding hypoglycaemia, and uncontrolled hyperglycaemia. Subsequently, management will be geared more towards the prevention and management of diabetes-related complications, with a heavy emphasis on reducing the risk of cardiovascular disease. Suitable education and support for the patient is vital in achieving these goals. Each person should have an individualized care plan that can be recorded and modified (50, see overleaf). Components included within this care plan should be:

❑ Diabetes education.
❑ Dietary advice.
❑ Insulin therapy.
❑ Self-monitoring.
❑ Vascular risk factor assessment.
❑ Late complications surveillance.
❑ Method and frequency of communication with the care team.
❑ Annual review.

Those with Type 1 diabetes require at least an annual assessment of education and skills relating to diet, lifestyle, glucose control, and insulin dose adjustment. There should also be an assessment of vascular risk factors and their treatment, i.e. blood pressure, lipid profile, and smoking habits for all diabetic patients. In addition, there should be an assessment of any complications (retinopathy, neuropathy, nephropathy, foot disease, vascular disease).

Long-term follow-up

Patients with Type 2 diabetes should be seen and assessed by someone with an interest in and knowledge of diabetes every 6 months. This should be weekly or monthly in patients who are newly diagnosed, who are failing to achieve goals, or who are receiving adjustments to medication. If there are active complications, the patient is unwell, or making changes in insulin treatment there may need to be daily contact. *Table 53* presents the components of the complete consultation for Type 2 diabetes.

Table 52 Situations for referring a patient to hospital care

❑ The patient is acutely unwell
❑ The patient has diabetes at a time of life that requires specific specialist input (i.e. childhood or adolescence diabetes, pregnancy)
❑ There are complications of diabetes at presentation that require specific management (e.g. foot ulceration, renal disease)
❑ There are additional specialist medical problems (e.g. a drug or endocrine cause for diabetes)
❑ The patient needs to be provided with additional focussed specialty input (e.g. dietitians, podiatrists, nurses, psychologists)
❑ The person looking after the patient does not have the adequate knowledge or skills to manage the patient (e.g. patient requires insulin)

Table 53 The complete Type 2 diabetes consultation

History:	Review patient's symptoms
	Assess other medical illnesses and complications
	Assess home blood glucose measurements
	Check medication and adherence/side-effects
	Assess frequency/severity of hypoglycaemia
	Check for other psychosocial issues
Examination:	Check weight
	Check blood pressure
	Examine feet
	Examine other medical problems
	Check fundi annually
	Physical examination annually
Investigations:	Annual HbA1c or fructosamine assay
	Annual renal function and electrolytes
	Annual lipid profile (fasting if reasonable)
	Annual urinalysis
	Annual assay for microalbuminuria
Management review:	Address glycaemic control and symptoms/hypoglycaemia
	Address complications
	Address cardiovascular risk factors (lipids, blood pressure, weight)
	Address lifestyle adjustments (diet, exercise, smoking)
	Annual assessment of diabetes knowledge/self-management
	Address psychosocial issues
	Establish realistic management goals, provide advice/support

50	
Standard (100% target)	**Exceptions**
1. Confirmation at diagnosis	None
2. a. Assessment of glycaemic control b. Management of sub-optimal glycaemic control (HbA1C 6.5–7.5% dependent upon CVS risk)	a. Asymptomatic patients where diabetes complications are less relevant e.g. terminally ill patients b. As 2a
3. a. Weight b. Management of obesity (BMI >30 kg/m^2)	a. As 2a b. As 2a
4. a. Blood pressure b. Treatment of hypertension (BP >130/75 to 140/85 mmHg – on 3 separate occasions dependent upon CVS risk	a. As 2a b. As 2a

5. a. Retinal screening
 	
   b. Management of retinopathy
	a. Type 1 DM <5 years duration
	   • <13 years old
	   • Registered blind
	   • Under active follow-up of Eye Department
	   • As 2a
	b. None

6. a. Foot screening
 	
   b. Management of at risk foot or established foot disease (neuropathy, vascular disease, ulceration, callus formation, the postoperative limb or baseline foot screen assessment score >25)
	a. Type 1DM <5 years duration
	   • <13 years old
	b. None

50 Shared care plan for the management of diabetes.

Action	Monitoring of standards
Confirmation of diagnosis using WHO criteria	Documentation of criteria for diagnosis
HbA1C Consideration of: • Dietary assessment in all cases (by dietician/appropriately trained health care professional) +/− psychological assessment • +/− oral hypoglycaemic agents (OHA) • +/− insulin	Documentation of HbA1C or reason for not monitoring Documentation of dietary advice and by whom OHA commenced or adjusted by primary/secondary care Insulin commenced (or adjusted) usually by secondary care Plans for subsequent monitoring
Standard recording • Dietary review (by dietician/appropriately trained health care professional) • Advice on physical activity/lifestyle • +/− drug therapy • +/− surgery	Recorded evidence of weight Documented advice given concerning diet/lifestyle/drugs/surgery
Standard recording. If high (see 4b) re-measure within 6 weeks Drug treatment implemented (if non-pharmacological measures unsuccessful/inappropriate)	Recorded evidence of measurement Recorded evidence of introduction of treatment and plans for subsequent monitoring
Minimum of annual direct fundoscopic examination (dilated pupils) by health care professional competent in screening for diabetic retinopathy and/or Retinal photography Any degree of retinopathy: at high vascular risk requiring optimal glucose and BP control Background retinopathy: reviews (max 9 months) Pre-proliferative/severe background: ophthalmology referral (soon) Proliferative eye disease: ophthalmology referral (urgent) Macular disease: ophthalmology referral (soon)	Documented objective evidence of retinal screening Documented evidence of attempts to optimise diabetes/blood pressure control Documented evidence of ophthalmic referral
Annual clinical examination of feet for evidence of callus, ulceration, neuropathy or impaired circulation May include foot advice from trained health care professional, podiatry input or referral via diabetes foot care pathway Any degree of neurovascular foot disease: at high vascular risk requiring optimal glucose and BP control	Recorded evidence of foot screen (ideally recorded using District foot screen form) Recorded evidence of advice/referral and appropriate investigations *(Continued overleaf)*

Figure **50** continued from previous page

Standard (100% target)	Exceptions
7. a. Assessment of renal function	a. Type 1 DM <5 years duration • <13 years old • As 2a
b. Management of clinical nephropathy (& Type 2 diabetes – ACR >3 if tested) Type 1 Diabetes – persistent ACR >3 Type 2 Diabetes – persistent proteinuria Either – Creatinine >150 µmol/l	b. None
8. a. Assessment of lipid status (3 yearly if normal, annually if abnormal)	a. • <18 years old • Within 3 months of diagnosis of diabetes • As 2a
b. Management of dyslipidaemia	b. As 2a
9. a. Assessment of macrovascular risk	a. As 2a
b. Management of macrovascular risk	b. As 2a
10.a. Pregnancy counselling for premenopausal females	a. None
b. Pregnancy (includes gestational diabetes)	b. None
11. Thyroid function testing	None
NB: These standards outline the minimum standards for annual screening although more frequent monitoring may be required in certain given clinical situations. For auditing purposes, evaluation of the previous 15 months is recommended to allow for missed/delayed appointments, etc	

Action	Monitoring of standards
• Serum creatinine • Type 1 (test for microalbuminuria) – ACR • Type 2 (routinely tested for proteinuria.) ACR as per GP contract (will only impact upon management if otherwise intermediate CVS risk) • At high vascular risk requiring optimal glucose and BP control • Introduction of ACE inhibitor • Referral to hospital diabetes team/nephrologists • Stop metformin if relevant	Recorded evidence of biochemical assessment Recorded evidence of management action
• Screen: random cholesterol measurement • Follow district guidelines for cholesterol testing and therapy choices (known formerly as LEAP guidelines) According to district guidelines on primary/secondary prevention • Excluded other secondary causes • Dietary advice (dietician/appropriately trained health care professional) • At high vascular risk requiring optimal glucose, lipid and BP control • Specific lipid lowering agents	Recorded evidence of lipid concentration(s) Recorded evidence of diet/lifestyle advice/drug intervention
• Assess vascular risk • Any 1 high risk parameter implies high vascular risk • Conventional cardiovascular investigation and management • Aggressive treatment of reversible risk factors • If in high vascular risk group introduce aspirin	Recorded evidence of assessment where appropriate • Recorded evidence of appropriate management e.g. ECG, exercise test, carotid dopplers, etc • Treatment with aspirin, anti-anginal agent, hospital referral, etc
• As soon as considered appropriate – advice on maternal assessment prior to attempting pregnancy • Folic acid supplementation • Telephone referral to hospital diabetes centre within 1 week of confirmation of pregnancy in pre-gestational or diagnosis of gestational diabetic mother	Documentation that advice given
Consider at each visit on clinical merit. Conventional medical treatment of hyper/hypothyroidism	Documentation of thyroid function tests

BLOOD GLUCOSE CONTROL AND MONITORING

The importance of optimal glucose control in Type 1 diabetes was confirmed in the Diabetes Control and Complications Trial (DCCT). This was a landmark, large-scale multicentre study, where patients with Type 1 diabetes were randomly allocated to receive conventional or intensive insulin therapy. The intensively-treated group had a one-third reduction in mean blood glucose compared to the conventional group. This improved control gave a reduction in microvascular complications of 35–75% over 6.5 years. The frequency of retinopathy, nephropathy, and neuropathy was reduced, as well as the progression of established retinopathy.

Although this study demonstrated that targeting and achieving improved glucose control has a significant impact on reducing the microvascular complications in Type 1 diabetes, it also led to a threefold increase of severe hypoglycaemia in the intensive group. The UKPDS in 1999 confirmed similar reductions in microvascular complications for patients with Type 2 diabetes in whom glucose levels were treated aggressively.

Urinary dipstick testing for glucose is unreliable since urine glucose is a delayed reflection of blood glucose, is subject to individual variability in renal thresholds, and is imprecise. In addition, urine dipstick testing cannot diagnose hypoglycaemia.

Blood glucose self-monitoring enables patients to identify hyperglycaemia and hypoglycaemia easily and to monitor the effects of diet, lifestyle, and insulin therapy on glucose control. This can enable the prediction of blood glucose concentration so that adjustments in treatment or other factors can be made, improving the possibility of good glucose control whilst minimizing the risks of hypoglycaemia.

There are large numbers of simple blood glucose meters available to suit individual needs (**51**). The meters read colour change in enzyme-impregnated dry-reagent strips, frequently coated with glucose oxidase and peroxidase, or electrical current in electrochemical strips. These strips can be expensive. They are purchased separately and are available on prescription. Most testing devices require blood from fingertips for self-monitoring (testing the sides of the fingertips tends to be less painful than the fleshy pulp). Most blood-testing devices employ a spring-loaded lancet. Devices have been developed to test from other sites such as the forearm but have not yet proven completely reliable. Newer devices do tend to require less blood volume than older devices and may,

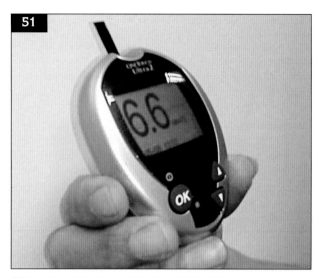

51 Insulin testing device: One Touch Ultra 2 meter.

therefore, be less uncomfortable. Low frequency of testing can be due to the discomfort associated with finger testing.

New watch devices have been developed to measure glucose concentration noninvasively (e.g. Glucowatch). These employ a technique called reverse iontophoresis. This involves the generation of a small current between electrodes resting on the surface of the skin. The electrical current draws fluid to the skin surface from which glucose is assayed. Problems with this technology include the need for prior calibration of the watch, local skin irritation, and device failure when there is excessive sweating. It can prove a useful tool for monitoring overnight glycaemic control and in other situations where multiple blood glucose values are required.

Glucose sensors for continuous monitoring of blood glucose are also becoming available. Minimally invasive sensors include needle electrodes and microdialysis probes implanted in subcutaneous tissue.

The frequency of self-monitoring will depend upon the individual's treatment regime, blood glucose control, individual lifestyle, and personal preference. Self-monitoring skills should be taught close to the time of diagnosis and initiation of insulin therapy. Self-monitoring skills, equipment, and the use of results should also be tested annually.

Blood glucose monitoring enables patients to examine the effects of insulin, diet, and lifestyle on

blood glucose so that appropriate adjustments can be learnt and implemented to improve blood glucose control. In addition, there are number of different circumstances where blood glucose self-monitoring becomes particularly important:
- During problematic hypoglycaemia or elevated blood sugars.
- During treatment changes.
- When exercise is being planned, is occurring, or has occurred.
- Changes in meal size and content or missed meals.
- Following alcohol consumption.
- During periods of ill-health.

Blood glucose measurements are probably most useful when taken prior to meal times, although 2-hour postprandial measurements give an idea of postprandial responses to different meal types. Serial timed blood glucose measurements are needed to give information that can be used to adjust insulin therapy. One-off measurements are generally unhelpful. Overnight measurements can be useful in determining whether there is nocturnal hypoglycaemia.

Preprandial blood glucose levels should ideally be 4–7 mmol/l and postprandial levels <9 mmol/l. However, tight blood glucose should not be pursued if the risk of hypoglycaemia is significant or quality of life is impaired. It is important to avoid the development of hypoglycaemic unawareness, suggested by undetected hypoglycaemic blood results.

HbA1c TESTING
In clinical practice the glycosylated haemoglobin (HbA1c) provides an objective measure of glucose control for the preceding 2–3 months. It is formed in the blood from nonenzymatic attachment of glucose to the N terminal end of the adult haemoglobin β-chain. There are different forms of glycosylated haemoglobin and there is significant variation between different laboratory results due to assay variations and the difficulty of standardization. Whichever form of glycosylated haemoglobin is measured, most laboratories are now aligned to the HbA1c method used in the DCCT study. At lower levels this approximates to mean plasma glucose concentration.

An HbA1c measurement enables clinicians to compare patterns of self-monitored blood glucose measurements with an objective measure of control. It should be measured every 6 months and more frequently when clinically indicated, for example during periods of treatment change or during pregnancy. The DCCT study demonstrated that the tighter the blood glucose control, the greater the reduction in microvascular complications. An HbA1c concentration of <6.5–7.5% should be targeted. In patients with additional cardiovascular risk, the lower threshold (<6.5%) should be the aim. Spuriously low HbA1c levels may be obtained in patients with a haemoglobinopathy, reduced red cell survival (e.g. haemolysis, bleeding), and the anaemia of renal failure. High levels of haemoglobin F can artificially elevate HbA1c levels.

An alternative measurement to HbA1c is a serum fructosamine. This is a measure of glycosylated serum proteins, mostly albumin. It gives an index of glucose control over the previous 2–3 weeks. It is used less frequently now but can be a useful measurement when a reflection of more recent blood glucose concentrations is required, e.g. during pregnancy, or where a haemoglobinopathy is present. The normal range for fructosamine in nondiabetic subjects is 205–285 µmol/l. Its values increase in a linear relationship to HbA1c (a serum fructosamine of 400 µmol/l corresponds to an HbA1c of about 9%).

MANAGING DIET IN TYPE 2 DIABETES
Healthy eating is an essential component of diabetes health care. Following a suitable diet can have a beneficial effect on weight, glucose control, and wellbeing. It can also reduce vascular risk through improving the lipid profile, lowering blood pressure, and reducing central obesity. Dietary counselling involves a number of different stages. These include an assessment of current diet and readiness for change, discussion of change, the setting of realistic patient-centred goals, and regular monitoring and support. Dietary advice is an area of enormous complexity and disagreement and this can cause confusion for patients and health care professionals.

When giving dietary advice balance needs to be struck between reducing the risk of disease complications and ensuring a healthy balance of food types and nutrients.

One simple agreed model for good health is 'The Balance of Good Health' (Leicestershire Health, 1997). This model divides food into five groups:
- Fruit and vegetables.
- Bread/cereal/potatoes.
- Dairy products.
- Meat/fish.
- Fatty/sugary foods.

It is recommended that those with Type 2 diabetes eat five portions of fruit and vegetables daily, eat five portions of high fibre bread/cereal/potatoes, eat lower fat dairy products including milk, eat a maximum of two portions of low fat meat/fish, and reduce intake of fatty or sugary food. Meals and snacks should be spaced appropriately throughout the day to avoid fluctuation in glycaemic control. In those who are overweight, dietary advice should aim for a reduced energy intake in order to facilitate weight loss. Patients should be advised to avoid the intake of foods that are energy-dense, particularly fatty foods and alcohol. It should be remembered that weight loss is not a normal physiological state and is, therefore, difficult and frequently unsuccessful

Carbohydrate

Carbohydrate ingested in the form of starch (complex carbohydrate) rather than sugars (fast-acting or simple carbohydrate) slows digestion and the rate at which glucose and other simple sugars enter the circulation. This reduces postprandial hyperglycaemia. The hyperglycaemic potential of different foods is sometimes expressed as the 'glycaemic index'. This is calculated from the proportion of glucose present in the circulation following an ingestion of 50 g of the food compared with 50 g of a pure glucose solution. Low glycaemic index foods (e.g. rice, pasta, cereals, potatoes) are complex carbohydrates recommended in the dietary management of those with diabetes. Complex carbohydrate and monounsaturated fat should, in combination, make up 60–70% of energy intake.

Artificial sweeteners are widely used in commercial food and beverages. They appear to be a safe nonnutrient alternative to sugars. Dietary fibre also slows the digestion of carbohydrate and absorption of sugars by trapping them within a fibrous matrix. Fibres are mostly indigestible plant polysaccharides. Fibre should form >30 g in a daily diet and can be achieved through eating plenty of vegetables and pulses. This may have the additional effect of improving the lipid profile. A diet rich in vegetables, fruit, and cereals should provide adequate amounts of both complex carbohydrate and fibre.

Fat

Reducing fat in the diet is likely to be effective in reducing long-term cardiovascular risk and, in the short-term, it also has the effect of reducing insulin resistance. Fat has more than double the energy density of carbohydrate or protein. Being able to recognize fatty foods and find alternatives to them is essential in order to alter the proportion of fat in the diet. Ideally fat should form less than 30% of daily energy intake. Saturated fat is the predominant component of animal fat and should form less than 10% of total daily energy intake. Polyunsaturated fatty acids are mainly derived from plant sources, e.g. linoleic acid, found in vegetable oil. Small amounts of polyunsaturated fish oils can reduce triglyceride concentrations and reduce platelet aggregation but large quantities can worsen glycaemic control.

For those consuming Indo-Asian diets, olive oil should be used instead of ghee, fat should be drained off after frying spices, and there should be a reduction in consumption of some other traditional dishes (e.g. samosas, bhajis, and puris).

Protein

Daily protein intake should form about 15% of total daily energy intake (0.8 g/kg/body weight/day). Fish and lean meat should be encouraged in moderation. Cereals, pulses, soya products. and tofu also contain large amounts of protein. Excessive protein intake should be particularly avoided in renal failure where a low-protein diet is sometimes recommended.

Alcohol

Those with Type 2 diabetes are advised to drink alcohol in moderation and not on an empty stomach. They should not exceed the maximum nationally recommended weekly intake (UK: 28 units/week for men and 21 units/week for women). Binge drinking should be avoided but there is evidence that small amounts of alcohol (e.g. one glass of wine per day) consumed regularly may reduce cardiovascular risk. For those taking hypoglycaemic medication (tablets or insulin) there may be an increased reduction in blood glucose for a period of up to 8–10 hours after consumption. However, in Type 2 diabetes this rarely causes significant hypoglycaemia. There is evidence that alcohol can contribute to both hypertriglyceridaemia and hypertension.

Salt

Most patients with Type 2 diabetes are predisposed to hypertension. It is important therefore that daily salt consumption should not exceed 3 g/day. Potassium chloride is an alternative substitute to table salt but care should be taken to avoid hyperkalaemia in patients with renal failure or those on potassium-sparing diuretics and angiotensin-converting enzyme (ACE) inhibitors.

Vitamins, minerals, and micronutrients

Provided there are no complicating medical conditions, a healthy balanced diet should provide adequate quantities of nutrients for most. Supplementation is generally required only in the malnourished, early and prepregnancy, or in proven deficiency states. There is limited evidence to suggest any benefit for oral antioxidants in diabetes.

EXERCISE

Regular aerobic exercise improves insulin sensitivity and glucose control in Type 2 diabetes. It also reduces body fat, helps maintain muscle mass, and improves the blood lipid profile. There is evidence that regular exercise improves physical and psychological wellbeing. It is an effective way to reduce the risk of cardiovascular disease, the most common cause of death in Type 2 diabetes. Regular exercise can reduce long-term mortality in people with diabetes by 50–60% (Table 54).

In contrast to Type 1 diabetes, exercise does not usually cause hypoglycaemia in those with Type 2 diabetes, despite having have beneficial effects on lowering blood glucose levels. For those at increased risk of developing Type 2 diabetes, exercise reduces the likelihood of progressing to diabetes. For those who do not regularly take exercise, it is important to recommend an exercise activity that is enjoyable. It needs to be tailored to the individual to ensure that it is appropriate for that person's attitudes and preferences. It should be practicable within a patient's social and cultural setting. Importantly, all patients should receive a medical assessment before being considered for an exercise programme. It may be this assessment that decides the appropriate form of exercise programme and whether initial investigations are required in advance of that recommendation.

Simple initial advice might be to incorporate moderate exercise into the daily schedule, such as an extra 30 minutes of brisk walking, cycling, or swimming each day. Patients should be advised that the intensity and duration of exercise should be increased gradually. Although the risk of hypoglycaemia is low, advice should include carrying glucose supplements and diabetes identification whilst participating in exercise. Fluid should be consumed regularly. Exercise periods should include warm-up and cool-down periods to prevent unnecessary injury. Those with Type 2 diabetes frequently suffer with overt or subclinical cardiovascular disease. If this is suspected then these patients should be properly evaluated with a baseline ECG and formal exercise treadmill testing.

Patients with active proliferative retinopathy or uncontrolled hypertension should avoid exercises that increase introthoracic pressure (isometric exercises such as 'weights'). These patients should also avoid exercise that increase systolic blood pressure and should carry out exercise that keeps the pulse rate at <70% of maximum (maximum heart rate can be calculated as 220 bpm minus age). Patients with peripheral neuropathy and/or impaired circulation to the feet should be careful to avoid exercise that causes recurrent trauma, to the toes in particular. Jogging and step exercises are not suitable for these patients. Swimming, cycling, and chair-based exercises are more appropriate.

Exercise advice should include an assessment of the impact of tablet and insulin treatment. Although hypoglycaemia is rare, it is best to avoid exercise when blood glucose levels are low or when injected insulin levels are at their peak, e.g. soon after administration

---

Table 54 Beneficial effects of exercise in Type 2 diabetes

❑ Improvement in insulin sensitivity and reduction in blood glucose concentration

❑ Increasing energy expenditure favours weight loss

❑ Reduction in body fat and maintenance of muscle mass. (This may reduce the lowering of metabolic rate during slimming and therefore promote longer-term weight loss)

❑ Reductions in triglyceride and LDL-cholesterol concentration. Increased HDL-cholesterol concentration

❑ Improvement in psychological well being

❑ Reduced risk of cardiovascular risk and improved mortality rates

of a quick-acting insulin. Patients should be made aware of the risk of hypoglycaemia and that exercise increases the rate of insulin absorption. There are increasing numbers of exercise programmes being developed for patients with cardiovascular disease, diabetes, and obesity. These enable many to exercise with safety. It is important that programmes ensure an appropriate level of individualized supervision. There should be a balanced programme involving aerobic and anaerobic exercise at least 3–5 times per week. Each individual should be set early goals to help in the initial phases of an exercise programme. The emphasis, however, should be on changing activity and exercise habits in the long-term.

SMOKING

Cigarette smoking is a major, modifiable risk factor for cardiovascular disease in those with and without diabetes. The combination of diabetes and smoking greatly enhances the risk of coronary, cerebral, and peripheral vascular disease. Smoking also increases the risk of developing microvascular complications of diabetes (nephropathy, neuropathy, and retinopathy). Smoking cessation can reduce the risk of stroke, coronary disease, and major peripheral arterial disease by up to 30%. It is, therefore, important to find ways of stopping patients with diabetes from smoking.

There are several important techniques that can help in smoking cessation:
- ❏ A brief (3 minute) piece of advice from a health care professional, incorporating information about the benefits of being a nonsmoker and the dangers of being a smoker and suggesting a date to stop (effective in 2%).
- ❏ Nicotine replacement therapy (NRT) in motivated quitters who smoke heavily (>10 cigarettes per day).
- ❏ Use of smoking cessation clinics for motivated quitters.
- ❏ Bupropion (Zyban) or nortryptiline antidepressants combined with a structured counselling programme.

Medical therapies are only useful in those who are willing to quit smoking. NRT is now available in patches, gum, inhaler, and nasal spray and helps with physical withdrawal symptoms. It is available on prescription or over the counter. The first prescription should be for 2 weeks after the stop date, but more should be prescribed if cessation is successful and symptoms persist. Bupropion (Zyban) should be prescribed for 3–4 weeks after the stop date. There is a small risk of seizures in susceptible individuals and it should only be prescribed for adults (>18 years).

EDUCATING ABOUT GLUCOSE CONTROL AND REDUCING RISK

It is important to explain to patients why they should aim for good glucose contol in the long-term. The DCCT and UKPDS studies have clearly identified that tight glucose control reduces the risk of microvascular complications of both Type 1 and Type 2 diabetes. Tissue damage appears to be related to the duration and severity of hyperglycaemia. There is also evidence that lower levels of blood glucose are associated with a reduction in cardiovascular disease and other circulatory events such as stroke. The UKPDS study also showed that improved glucose control is difficult to achieve in Type 2 diabetes. Despite intensive follow-up and increased combination therapy, the intensively treated group achieved a mean HbA1c of 7.0% compared to 7.9% in the conservatively managed group. However, this small improvement in HbA1c did confer a benefit. The benefit of lowering blood glucose continues to accrue until normal levels of blood glucose are achieved. Excessively rigorous efforts to normalize blood glucose may, however, significantly increase the risk of hypoglycaemia.

Although most patients will require drug therapy within 3 years of being diagnosed with Type 2 diabetes, there is usually a drop in blood glucose at diagnosis that can be maintained without drug therapy. This can be helped through lifestyle adjustments described extensively in this chapter.

The aims of glucose control are threefold in both Type 1 and Type 2 diabetes:
- ❏ Avoiding hypoglycaemia (in those on medication only).
- ❏ Achieving normoglycaemia (preprandial or fasting glucose concentration of 4–7 mmol/l).
- ❏ Avoiding hyperglycaemia (an HbA1c of <6.5–7.5%; the lower value should be targeted for those at highest cardiovascular risk).

Patients should be educated to recognize warning signs of hypoglycaemia and understand the impact of lifestyle, meals, and exercise. Where appropriate they should be educated in finger-prick capillary blood glucose monitoring and how to interpret and adjust to these results and those of laboratory HbA1c measurements.

DRIVING AND DIABETES

All those with diabetes that is controlled by tablets or insulin should report their condition to the DVLA. The patient should also inform the DVLA of any diabetes complications or visual problems that could impair their ability to drive. Visual standards that need to be achieved are a corrected Snellen chart visual acuity of 6/12 and a visual field of 120° in the horizontal axis and 20° in the vertical axis. Patients who are commenced on insulin therapy need to inform the DVLA immediately of this change of therapy. Driving requirements for patients taking insulin are stricter. Ordinary (Group 1) licence holders have to demonstrate 'satisfactory' control and be able to recognize symptoms of hypoglycaemia. They will be given a licence for a period of 1–3 years and this will then be reviewed. Medical confirmation is frequently requested. Those taking insulin are banned from holding a Group 2 licence, required for driving a bus, coach, or large goods vehicle. Patients breaching these regulations run the risk of being charged with 'driving under the influence of drugs'.

TRAVEL

Patients with diabetes are free to travel. Planning for travel is essential, particularly for those patients who receive insulin treatment. Medication and diabetes equipment should be accessible throughout the journey. It should be stored in hand luggage and not stowed in the hold of a plane. Prescription tablets should be kept in their original containers and equipment kept in plastic bags with zipper seals. Insulin should be kept away from heat and direct sunlight and stored in a cool bag where possible. Patients should carry medical identification and a headed letter from a doctor or nurse, listing the medication and devices that they require.

Adequate medication should be taken for the trip. If this is not possible, checks should be made for the availability of tablets and insulin abroad. For those on insulin therapy, it is important to ensure that U100 insulin is used in the destination country. If only U40 insulin is available, this should be taken via U40 syringes to avoid dosing mistakes. It is important to remain well hydrated by consuming plenty of water or energy-free fluid during the journey. Carbohydrate should continue to be ingested to reduce the risk of hypoglycaemia. Those on medication should always continue treatment.

When crossing time zones, insulin treatment requires alteration. Typically, there should be a reduction in background insulin dose to avoid hypoglycaemia. More emphasis is then placed on short-acting insulin, taken with each meal, to control blood glucose. Perfect glucose control is difficult to achieve during travel and the aim is to avoid hypoglycaemia and severe hyperglycaemia. This usually results in higher than usual blood glucose during the period of travel. It is important to monitor frequently, where possible. A local professional or service can provide printed recommendations or individualized dosage change advice. Additional help can be obtained from the Diabetes UK website.

Those with diabetes should be aware that heat can increase the rate of insulin absorption and also lead to dehydration. Dietary and exercise patterns may also be different. Regular self-monitoring and insulin dose adjustment, together with regular consumption of water should reduce the risk of hypo- and hyperglycaemia. Foot complications are more common during travel. At-risk patients should avoid going barefoot and check that shoes are well fitting. It is important that those with diabetes ensure they have adequate health insurance cover for travel.

INSURANCE

Diabetes may lead to higher premiums for car, travel, and life insurance quotes but it is essential to shop around. Diabetes UK provides car insurance but this may not necessarily be the cheapest.

RELIGION AND DIABETES

Professionals helping those with diabetes should ensure that they are providing equal access to and are equally responsive to people from all social, ethnic, and cultural backgrounds. They should be aware that diet, lifestyle, and health beliefs vary enormously and their management should be tailored to take these considerations into account.

Ramadan is a religious period that requires specific adaptation of diabetes treatment. During this month, healthy Moslem adults will usually fast between dawn and sunset. Two meals are usually consumed, at the end of the day and early the following morning. These meals may be rich in carbohydrate. It may be helpful to advise limiting carbohydrate-rich and fatty foods. Metformin should be taken at the end of the fast before the evening meal. It may need to be reduced or stopped. Quick-acting sulphonylureas are recommended. These are probably best taken before the morning meal.

PHARMACOLOGICAL TREATMENT IN TYPE 1 DIABETES

Insulin is required in all patients with Type 1 diabetes. It is typically given by the subcutaneous route although inhaled quick-acting preparations are now available. Insulin is available in vials, 3 ml cartridges for pen injection devices, and disposable pen devices. Insulin is mostly produced in a biosynthetic form. Animal insulins are now being mostly phased out. Side-effects of insulin are weight gain and hypoglycaemia

Juggling the effects of insulin administration and lifestyle factors on glucose control is a lifetime project for the patient with Type 1 diabetes. The timing and content of meals, the effects of alcohol, exercise, and ill health on glucose control may lead to changes in insulin doses or even regimes on a regular basis. Patients should be educated about the effects of lifestyle factors on insulin requirements. The location of injection sites, ambient temperature, and other factors that relate to the administration of insulin can also impact on glucose control. The choice of insulin regime and insulin types should be made jointly by the patient and health care professional and will be affected by practical issues such as variability of lifestyle and ease of use of injection tools. Initiation of insulin therapy should be accompanied by initiation of blood glucose monitoring in addition to a full educational package of care.

TYPES OF INSULIN

Traditional shorter-acting (soluble) insulin preparations, e.g. human actrapid, have an onset 30 minutes after injection and a duration of 6–8 hours with a peak onset of 2–4 hours. They should be injected 20–30 minutes before eating a meal. Quick-acting insulin analogues, e.g. Insulin Lyspro and Insulin Aspart, have a more rapid onset, earlier peak effect, and shorter duration of action so can be given immediately before a meal. Traditional longer-acting (intermediate or isophane) insulin preparations, e.g. Humulin I or Insulatard, have an onset of action 1–2 hours after injection, a peak of 4–6 hours and a duration up to 14 hours. Basal insulin analogues, e.g. Insulin Glargine and Insulin Determir, are long-acting basal analogues that have a loger duration of action and a more 'peakless' profile than traditional longer-acting insulins, i.e. the basal level of insulin provided is more stable leading to less of a peak with a reduced risk of hypoglycaemia.

Mixed insulin preparations contain a combination of a shorter-acting (or quick-acting analogue insulin) and an intermediate insulin, e.g. Mixtard 30, Humulin M3, Novomix 30, Humalog Mix25. These combine the properties of the different insulin types and are usually administered twice daily prior to breakfast and evening meal.

In continuous subcutaneous insulin infusion (CSII), soluble insulin is given subcutaneously through a cannula implanted subcutaneously. This allows for continuous delivery of insulin with an increased rate delivered at the time of eating. Early problems with infections and pump failure are now much less common. The major problem with this form of treatment is cost. Pumps and consumable materials are prohibitively expensive (**52**).

Inhaled insulin (Exubera and others forthcoming) are very expensive but a form of insulin administration that might be preferred by patients. These inhaled forms of insulin can replace the shorter-acting component of an insulin regime so are unlikely to replace the need for injections altogether. There is still uncertainty over long-term safety and they are not recommended for smokers or those with acute or chronic respiratory disease. Regular measurement of vital capacity is currently required following initiation of therapy since there are reports of respiratory impairment in some patients. These patients should not remain on this therapy. Traditional commonly-used insulin preparations are listed in *Table 55*.

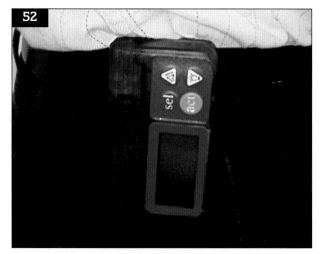

52 Insulin pump: Minimed 508 pump.

Table 55 Insulin preparations

Shorter-acting	Longer-acting	Mixed
Actrapid	Insulatard	Mixtard range
Humulin S	Humulin S	Humulin M range
Insulin Lyspro (analogue)	Glargine (basal analogue)	Humalog Mix 25 (includes analogue)
Aspart (analogue)	Determir (basal analogue)	NovoMix 30
Insuman		

INSULIN REGIMES

Twice daily regimes

For twice daily regimes, a typical starting dose of a mixed insulin preparation is recommended, although short- and long-acting insulins can be coadministered to increase flexibility of dosage. A starting dose of a premixed insulin might be 8 units twice daily (**53**). The aim should be for half to two-thirds of the total daily dose to be given at breakfast and one-third to a half with the evening meal. There are now easily accessible insulin titration regimes to enable rapid, safe increases of insulin dose until appropriate glycaemic control is achieved. Where it is felt there may be benefit, mixed preparations that incorporate a rapid-acting analogue are available. This allows patients to inject immediately before meals. With traditional mixed insulins or with combinations of traditional short- and long-acting preparations, insulin should be administered 20–30 minutes prior to eating.

Basal bolus regimes

Some patients may prefer the basal bolus system of insulin administration (**54**). It allows for flexibility of dose adjustment and can also be useful in those who require large doses of insulin. Often it is younger patients or those with more day-to-day variation of eating and lifestyle patterns that benefit most from a basal bolus system of insulin administration. This system allows individuals to give insulin more effectively according to their dietary and exercise requirements for that day. The advent of rapid-acting insulin analogues also allows insulin to be administered immediately prior to a meal rather than 20–30 minutes beforehand. These newer analogues also reduce the need for frequent snacking since they exit the system as quickly as they arrive.

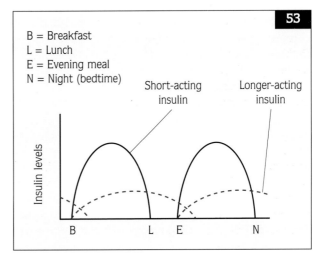

53 Diagram to illustrate insulin levels in the twice daily (b.d.) insulin regime.

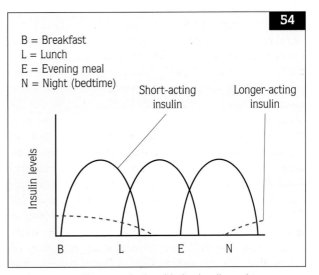

54 Diagram to illustrate the basal bolus insulin regime.

Using a basal bolus system a long-acting or long-acting analogue insulin is administered once daily, most commonly prior to bedtime. This provides the basal insulin requirements. Quick-acting insulin is given prior to meals and/or snacks to cover glycaemic excursions occurring as a result of food intake.

PHARMACOLOGICAL TREATMENT IN TYPE 2 DIABETES
ORAL HYPOGLYCAEMIC AGENTS

Pharmacological treatment to lower blood glucose in patients with Type 2 diabetes is recommended when dietary and lifestyle adjustment fails to achieve or maintain adequate glycaemic control. There are several different classes of antidiabetic drugs currently available. The major therapies used are:
❑ Metformin.
❑ Thiazolidinediones.
❑ Sulphonylureas.
❑ Meglitidine analogues.
❑ α-glucosidase inhibitors.
❑ Insulin.

Metformin and the thiazolidinediones (currently rosiglitazone and pioglitazone) are insulin-sensitizing agents. The sulphonylurea drugs and meglitidines stimulate insulin secretion from the pancreas gland. The α-glucosidase inhibitors reduce intestinal absorption of sugars.

Since the 1950s when the first sulphonylurea drugs and the first biguanides were introduced, these two classes of drug have dominated the oral hypoglycaemic marketplace. Recently the introduction of the α-glucosidase inhibitors in the early 1990s, the meglitidine analogues in the late 1990s and, most dramatically, the thiazolidinediones in the late 1990s, have complicated the oral management of Type 2 diabetes. Despite their dominance, both the sulphonylurea drugs and the biguanides have had a chequered and controversial history. In the 1970s phenformin was discontinued due to worries about the increased risk of lactic acidosis, leaving metformin as the only remaining biguanide. At around the same time, the University Group Diabetes Program (UGDP) raised worries about potentially damaging cardiovascular effects of the sulphonylurea drugs. These concerns have not been backed up by further studies or clinical experience. The UKPDS study group failed to find any difference in mortality or morbidity of patients taking metformin, the sulphonylurea drug glibenclamide, or insulin as first-line therapy. In a subgroup of overweight patients, however, intensive first-line therapy with metformin led to a reduction in mortality and MI compared with conventional therapy. This has led to a general acceptance that metformin should be used as first-line oral therapy in overweight patients with Type 2 diabetes. This finding supports what was already a trend emerging in diabetes management.

There is now evidence emerging from thiazolidinedione studies that this group of agents may be important in patients with the insulin resistance syndrome that make up a large proportion of those with Type 2 diabetes. We await the results of studies that might indicate whether these perceived benefits place them ahead of other therapies in the oral management of Type 2 diabetes.

The traditional order of tablet management in Type 2 diabetes may be changing but a common order of management for an overweight patient is as follows:
1. Commence metformin following failure of diet and lifestyle.
2. Following titration to maximum dose of metformin, introduce a sulphonylurea drug.
3. Following maximal titration of sulphonylurea, consider adding in a thiazolidinedione.
4. Consider other agents such as acarbose or appetite suppressants, re-explore diet and lifestyle.
5. Consider the introduction of insulin therapy, often continuing metformin but discontinuing other therapies.

Metformin

French lilac is a guanidine-containing product that has been used historically as a treatment for diabetes. Guanidine has a blood glucose-lowering effect. In the 1950s, metformin, phenformin, and buformin were introduced. Phenformin was withdrawn from most countries due to a high incidence of lactic acidosis associated with the drug. Buformin has never been widely used. Metformin, however, is now the most commonly prescribed oral hypoglycaemic worldwide.

Metformin is a stable hydrophilic biguanide. It is excreted unchanged in the urine and should be avoided in patients with significant renal tubular impairment to avoid accumulation of the drug. It is distributed in most tissues, but particularly the gastrointestinal tract. It is not protein-bound and 90% of the drug is eliminated within 12 hours. Metformin acts partly by improving insulin action and partly through mechanisms that do not depend upon insulin. Metformin lowers blood glucose concentration without causing hypoglycaemia. It does not stimulate insulin release from the pancreas. In fact, it typically causes a slight reduction in plasma insulin concentration.

Its most potent effect is its reduction of hepatic glucose production. It reduces hepatic gluconeogenesis primarily by increasing hepatic sensitivity to insulin. It also opposes the effects of glucagon and reduces hepatic glycogenolysis. Metformin enhances insulin-stimulated glucose uptake and glycogen formation in skeletal muscle by increasing the number of glucose transporters in the cell membrane and increasing the activity of glycogen synthase. At cellular level, the glucose-lowering effect of metformin relates predominantly to an increase of insulin-stimulated tyrosine kinase signalling activity of the insulin receptor. Metformin also suppresses fatty acid oxidation and reduces triglyceride levels in patients with hypertriglyceridaemia.

Metformin has traditionally been the treatment of choice for overweight patients with Type 2 diabetes because it does not lead to weight gain. It is also effective in those Type 2 patients who are not over-weight. It is now a first-line treatment for most Type 2 patients who have failed to achieve adequate glycaemic control with diet and lifestyle modification. It can be used alone, where it does not cause hypoglycaemia, or in combination with other oral hypoglycaemic agents and insulin. It has also been shown to be effective in restoring menstrual cycle and fertility in women with anovulatory polycystic ovarian syndrome (PCOS).

Metformin should not be started in patients with significantly impaired renal function (serum creatinine >130 μmol/l) to prevent drug accumulation, cardiac failure, severe respiratory disease, sepsis, or any other condition that predisposes to tissue hypoxia. It should also be avoided in patients with liver disease, alcoholism, or a history of metabolic acidosis. Metformin should be taken immediately before meals to minimize the possibility of gastro-intestinal side-effects. The tablet should be started at a dose of 500–850 mg once a day or 500 mg twice daily with morning and evening meals. The dose can be altered at 2-weekly intervals depending upon blood glucose response. A dose increase should be by one tablet (500–850 mg) at a time. The most effective dose is usually 2000 mg/day. If an increase in dose produces no beneficial effect on blood glucose, then it

should be reduced to the previous dose and combination therapy should be considered. There are now commercially available combinations of metformin with a sulphonylurea and metformin with a thiazolidinedione. There is also a slow release metformin preparation now available.

Side-effects from metformin are mainly gastro-intestinal and are strongly dose-related. Diarrhoea and abdominal discomfort are commonplace during the introduction of metformin. In fact it is not uncommon to find patients on metformin receiving unnecessary extensive gastrointestinal investigation because of troublesome drug-related symptoms. Symptoms usually abate if the drug is reduced or stopped and then re-introduced gradually. An asymptomatic dose can be found in 90–95% of patients.

Metformin can cause vitamin B12 deficiency in those with a poor diet since it impairs gastrointestinal absorption of this vitamin. It is, therefore, worth checking both a full blood count and renal function annually. Metformin should be stopped during the use of intravenous radiographic contrast media or surgery due to the potential risk of lactic acidosis. It can increase the risk of hypoglycaemia when used in combination with other hypoglycaemic agents.

Beneficial effects of metformin

The glucose-lowering effect of metformin is similar to that of the sulphonylurea drugs. It reduces HbA1c by 1–2% and fasting plasma glucose (FPG) by 2–4 mmol/l in patients poorly controlled on diet. It is effective in all patient types but does depend on some residual β-cell function.

The main advantages of metformin are that it does not cause hypoglycaemia when used alone and it is weight neutral, or marginally weight-reducing. It also improves the lipid profile through a fall in triglyceride and low-density lipoprotein (LDL)-cholesterol and an increase in high-density lipoprotein (HDL)-cholesterol. In the UKPDS study, overweight patients treated aggressively and started on metformin had a significantly reduced risk of MI.

Combining metformin with all other oral hypoglycaemic agents leads to a fall in blood glucose provided there is residual β-cell function. Combining metformin with insulin therapy leads to a reduction in insulin dose to maintain normoglycaemia. Combining metformin with insulin, therefore, has the additional benefit of less hypoglycaemia and less insulin-induced weight gain.

Adverse effects of metformin

Lactic acidosis is the most serious side-effect associated with metformin. It is, however, astonishingly rare (about 1 in 30 000 users) and is restricted to case reports. The background incidence of lactic acidosis is not known but the condition has a 50% mortality rate. Since renal failure causes accumulation of the drug it should be withdrawn in those with renal failure, e.g. creatinine >150 μmol/l. Metformin should be stopped in all patients with suspected lactic acidosis (decreased pH <7.25, raised anion gap >15 mmol/l, and raised blood lactate >5 mmol/l). Treatment of lactic acidosis is with intravenous bicarbonate, correction of any hypoxia, and treatment of the underlying condition. Circulating metformin can also be removed by haemodialysis if levels are elevated (>5 μmol/l).

The thiazolidinediones

The thiazolidinediones are frequently termed TZDs or 'glitazones'. The first TZD to become commercially available was troglitazone which was introduced to the US market in 1997. It was withdrawn in 2000 due to reports of fatal hepatotoxicity. Two newer TZDs have been introduced that do not have an association with this serious side-effect, rosiglitazone and pioglitazone. These agents improve insulin sensitivity by stimulating a nuclear receptor known as peroxisome proliferator activated receptor-gamma. They are therefore also referred to as PPARγ agonists. Rosiglitazone and pioglitazone are both absorbed quickly with a peak circulatory concentration reached within 2 hours. Both drugs are metabolized by the liver. Rosiglitazone is predominantly excreted in the urine, pioglitazone's more active metabolites are mostly excreted in bile. Rosiglitazone is metabolized by CYP2C8, pioglitazone is partly metabolized by isoforms of cytochrome P450. However, no drug interactions have been reported. Both are mostly bound to plasma proteins and are at low concentrations.

TZDs stimulate PPARγ which is mostly found in adipose tissue where it helps to increase the transcription of insulin-sensitive genes such as GLUT-4, lipoprotein lipase, and several others. Stimulation of PPARγ by a TZD enhances sensitivity to insulin and increases lipogenesis. PPARγ is also found in skeletal muscle and liver where it enhances the action of insulin, increasing glucose uptake in muscle via GLUT-4 and reducing gluconeogenesis in the liver. Stimulation of lipogenesis by TZDs also reduces circulating nonesterified fatty acid (NEFA) concentrations.

There are also reductions in serum insulin, circulating triglyceride, and tumour necrosis factor-α (TNF-α). These changes also increase insulin sensitivity. TZDs require the presence of insulin to activate their genes and generate significant glucose-lowering effects. This effect is predominantly linked to their lipogenic activity. Rosiglitazone and pioglitazone can be used alone or in combination with either metformin or a sulphonylurea drug. Rosiglitazone and pioglitazone are available for use as monotherapy in the US but have been indicated only for use in combination with metformin or a sulphonylurea drug in Europe.

Despite a number of potential advantages, the current National Institute of Clinical Excellence (NICE) guidance (August 2003) recommends that a TZD be used as second-line therapy to either metformin or a sulphonylurea drug only in patients who are unable to tolerate a metformin and sulphonylurea combination or where either drug is contraindicated. This position has caused controversy and may change in the future. For many, an indication for commencing a TZD in the UK has been inadequate glycaemic control on monotherapy (frequently metformin) in an obese patient who exhibits features of the insulin resistance syndrome.

Rosiglitazone should be started at 2 mg once or twice per day and titrated up to a maximum of 8 mg/day. Pioglitazone should be started at 15 mg once per day and titrated up to 45 mg/day. Both can be given as once daily preparations. The glucose-lowering effect of TZDs is gradual with the full effect not achieved until 6–10 weeks. It is important to wait 8 weeks before a dose increase. The TZDs can lead to fluid retention and increased plasma volume and decrease in haemoglobin concentration and haematocrit. There is a risk of oedema and anaemia. Patients with cardiac failure, significant peripheral oedema, anaemia, or impaired liver function should not receive this class of drug.

It is recommended that liver function is checked at baseline and at every 2 months for the first year. If liver enzymes increase significantly (>1.5 × baseline) the TZD should be discontinued. As experience and confidence has increased with the use of these drugs, many centres are now checking liver function with less regularity.

Early studies examining the glucose-lowering efficacy of TZDs indicated an HbA1c reduction of only 0.6%, but a number of these trials were of short duration. The maximal effect of TZDs takes longer than other agents because much of its efficacy occurs at nuclear level, increasing the expression of insulin-sensitive genes. It is likely that the glucose-lowering effect is greater than the early efficacy trials suggest. Subsequent studies carried out in combination with sulphonylureas and metformin suggest an average HbA1c reduction of about 1%. The TZDs appear to enhance both insulin sensitivity and endogenous β-cell activity.

Beneficial effects of TZDs

Much of the interest in TZDs stems from their effects on other metabolic factors that relate to insulin sensitivity. They appear to have a beneficial effect on a number of factors associated with cardiovascular disease. This includes a reduction in micro-albuminuria, hypertension, dyslipidaemia, visceral fat, prothrombotic plasminogen activator inhibitor-1 (PAI-1) and C-reactive protein. Large scale clinical outcome studies are required to determine whether they can impact on disease progression and cardiovascular events.

The UKPDS study showed an inevitable decline in the glucose control of patients with Type 2 diabetes despite ever increasing therapy. There is recent evidence from long-term data collection that the glucose-lowering effects of TZDs may be longer than traditional agents. There also evidence from animal studies that β-cell function is preserved. However, long-term studies are needed to verify whether long-term preservation of β-cell function in adults with Type 2 diabetes is a realistic prospect with TZD therapy.

Adverse effects of TZDs

Weight gain has been observed during TZD therapy. This is typically 2–3 kg over the first 12 months of use and is predominantly due to an increase in subcutaneous fat. The damaging visceral fat associated with increased cardiovascular risk is reduced.

Mild hypoglycaemia can occur if used alone, but TZDs can potentiate the hypoglycaemic effects of other drugs. The complications of peripheral oedema and mild anaemia are common. Exacerbation of cardiac failure, significant anaemia, and liver toxicity are rare but recognized associations. It is not known whether TZDs and their effect on the PPARγ expressed by many tissues will have other systemic effects on dividing cells or immune function, but recent experience has not highlighted any significant concerns.

The sulphonylureas

The sulphonylurea drugs stimulate the secretion of insulin from pancreatic β-cells to give a direct hypoglycaemic effect. They have been used extensively since the late 1950s in the treatment of Type 2 diabetes. The early agents, tolbutamide and carbutamide, were followed by chlorpropamide, acetohexamide, and tolazamide. Stronger second-generation sulphonylureas, glibenclamide, gliclazide, and glipizide, were produced in the 1970s and 1980s. Glimepiride emerged in the mid 1990s. The suphonylureas vary in their rates of metabolism, chemical activity, and rates of excretion. They are all absorbed quickly and reach a peak plasma concentration within 2–4 hours. Chlorpropamide has a long duration of action (>24 hours).

Glipizide and tolbutamide have a short duration of action (<12–15 hours). They are metabolized by the liver and are excreted in bile and urine. They are highly protein-bound and, when administered with other protein-bound drugs, e.g. warfarin, aspirin, and sulphonamides, the risk of hypoglycaemia is increased. Other drugs that potentiate the hypoglycaemic effects of sulphonylureas include alcohol, monoamine oxidase inhibitors, and fibrates.

Sulphonylureas bind to sulphonylurea receptors on pancreatic β-cells. This closes adenosine triphosphate (ATP) sensitive potassium (K^+) channels and causes depolarization of the cell membrane. This leads to an influx of calcium into the cell, and activates proteins that control the release of insulin granules. Sulphonyl-ureas may also potentiate insulin release through receptors on insulin granules and through activation of protein kinase C. These drugs can initiate first- and second-phase insulin release even when glucose concentrations are low and can cause hypoglycaemia.

The sulphonylurea drugs are a commonly used first-line therapy for Type 2 patients who have not achieved adequate glycaemic control through diet and lifestyle changes. They are no longer preferred as first-line therapy in patients who are overweight because they induce weight gain and, unlike metformin, have not been shown to reduce the risk of cardiovascular disease. The sulphonylureas can be used in combination with any of the other glucose-lowering therapies. They are commonly used in combination with metformin. They can be coprescribed with insulin but small advantages in insulin dose reduction confer no obvious benefit.

Shorter-acting preparations should be used in

patients who are elderly or at increased risk of hypoglycaemia. The starting dose should always be low (e.g. gliclazide 40 mg once or twice daily) and should be titrated upwards by 40–80 mg doses every 2 weeks in response to blood glucose measurements. If hypoglycaemia occurs, the new dose should be reduced to the previous dose. Glycaemic control can be verified with an HbA1c measurement). If glycaemic control is not achieved with a maximum dose of sulphonylurea (e.g. gliclazide 160 mg twice daily), additional oral agents can be added.

Beneficial effects of sulphonylureas
Sulphonylureas are effective glucose-lowering drugs. If treatment is titrated to the maximum dose it leads to a reduction in HbA1c of 1–2%. This effect is similar in most patient types but does depend on adequate β-cell function. Type 2 diabetes leads to β-cell failure and therapy increases over time. Current evidence suggests that this effect is independent of the drug used (i.e. sulphonylurea or metformin). There is some evidence that those prescribed newer sulphonylurea drugs may experience less rapid deterioration in glycaemic control than older agents. Early use of sulphonylureas is indicated when a single agent does not achieve adequate glucose control. The longer the delay in initiating sulphonylurea therapy, the less likely it is to prove effective. Sulphonylureas have a minimal effect on the lipid profile. The newer sulphonylurea agent glimepiride can be taken once daily and appears to have a lower incidence of hypoglycaemia and weight gain. The new once daily slow-release gliclazide preparation may have similar benefits.

Adverse effects of sulphonylureas
The sulphonylurea drugs cause weight gain of up to 4 kg over the first 6 months due to increased insulin secretion and reduced renal glucose excretion. This can be a significant problem in a population already struggling to lose weight. Of patients taking sulphonylurea therapy, 20% suffer from hypoglycaemia each year. Severe hypoglycaemia (defined as requiring assistance from a third party or requiring medical assistance) occurs in 1% of patients taking sulphonylureas each year. Hypoglycaemia is more likely in patients taking a longer acting sulphonylurea drug. Hypoglycaemia requires an assessment of drug choice, diet and exercise patterns, alcohol consumption, drug interactions, and intercurrent illness.

Other than hypoglycaemia and weight gain, side-effects can include a transient rash, rarely erythema multiforme, blood dyscrasias, fever, or jaundice. Chlorpropamide can lead to facial flushing after the ingestion of alcohol. It can also cause hyponatraemia. (It is occasionally used in the treatment of diabetes insipidus since it sensitizes renal tubules to the effect of antidiuretic hormone [ADH].) The sulphonylurea drugs should be used cautiously in patients with renal or liver disease.

The meglitidine analogues

The meglitidine analogues stimulate the first phase of insulin release that is lost in the early stages of Type 2 diabetes. Derivatives of meglitinide, a nonsulphonyl-urea, benzamido portion of glibenclamide, include repaglinide and nateglinide. These were introduced in the late 1990s. When taken immediately before a meal, they lead to an initial surge of insulin release that suppresses hepatic glucose output and reduces postprandial hyperglycaemia. Repaglinide is absorbed rapidly with peak plasma concentrations achieved in less than an hour. It is rapidly metabolized by the liver and excreted in bile. Its effect lasts only 3 hours. Nateglinide has a slightly faster rate of onset and a shorter duration of action.

Like the sulphonylurea drugs, the meglitidine analogues bind to sulphonylurea receptors on β-cells but bind closer to the ATP K⁺ channels. These agents should be taken 15–30 minutes before each main meal. The dose should be titrated slowly (repaglinide 0.5–4 mg/meal) with fortnightly increases in dose. If hypoglycaemia occurs then the prior dose should be used. HbA1c reductions of 1–2% are reported for repaglinide monotherapy. The meglitidine analogues can be used in combination with other oral hypoglycaemic agents with the exception of sulphony-lureas with which there is no additional benefit.

The indication for the meglitidine analogues is similar to that for the sulphonylureas but they may be more appropriate for those with postprandial hyperglycaemia or for those who have an erratic eating schedule. When used alone or in conjunction with metformin, this is likely to reduce the risk of hypoglycaemia compared with sulphonylureas. For these drugs to be effective there needs to be adequate β-cell function. There is likely to be some weight gain but no change in lipid profile. They should be used in caution in patients with liver or severe renal disease. Other than hypoglycaemia and weight gain, side-effects are rare. These drugs may interact with erythromycin, rifampicin, and antifungal agents.

Acarbose

Inhibitors of intestinal α-glucosidase enzymes reduce the rate of intestinal glucose absorption. This has the effect of reducing postprandial hyperglycaemia. Acarbose was introduced in the early 1990s. The α-glucosidase inhibitors inhibit the activity of these enzymes located in the brush border of gut enterocytes. This prevents the breakdown of disaccharides and oligosaccharides (e.g. sucrose and maltose) into absorbable monosaccharides. The effect is to delay and spread out intestinal glucose absorption. This reduces postprandial glucose concentration and secondarily insulin secretion. Acarbose should be taken with meals that contain digestible carbohydrate. It can be used as first-line monotherapy in patients with postprandial hyperglycaemia. It can also be used in combination with other oral glucose-lowering therapies and insulin. In monotherapy, it can lead to an HbA1c reduction of 1%. It does not cause weight gain and is associated with a slight lowering of serum triglyceride concentration. The use of acarbose is limited by tolerability that can be as low as 40%.

Gastrointestinal side-effects include flatulence, abdominal discomfort, and diarrhoea. These side-effects are common, particularly during the titration phase, so it is vital to titrate the dose very gradually and to ensure that the diet is rich in complex carbohydrate. The starting dose should be as low as 25–50 mg and is taken with the first mouthful of the main meal. Acarbose can be titrated up to 150 mg three times daily. Side-effects are typically dose-related but often settle over the course of a few days. Patients can be given a self-titration leaflet to help with dose titration. Acarbose should be avoided in patients with a history of gastrointestinal disturbance. Acarbose can also increase liver enzymes and these should be monitored and the dose reduced if the enzymes are elevated. It should not be prescribed in patients with liver or severe renal impairment.

NEWER GLUCOSE-LOWERING THERAPIES

Glucose homeostasis is dependent on a complex interplay of multiple hormones: insulin and amylin, produced by pancreatic β-cells; glucagon, produced by pancreatic α-cells; and gastrointestinal peptides including glucagon-like peptide-1 (GLP-1) and gastric inhibitory peptide (GIP). Abnormal regulation of these substances may contribute to the clinical presentation of diabetes. New drugs targeting these hormones have now been developed and can be used to help lower blood glucose levels. Pramlintide and exenatide have actions similar to amylin and GLP-1, respectively. These include delaying gastric emptying, regulating postprandial glucagon secretion, and reducing food intake. In addition, exenatide enhances glucose-dependent insulin secretion.

Pramlintide is an amylin analogue that is administered by mealtime subcutaneous injection. In the US its use has been approved for both Type 1 and insulin-treated Type 2 diabetes. It regulates postmeal blood glucose levels by slowing gastric emptying and suppressing the abnormal postprandial rise of glucagon in patients with diabetes. It does not cause hypoglycaemia. In Type 1 and insulin-treated Type 2 diabetes, pramlintide administered subcutaneously with meals results in reductions in HbA1c and modest reductions in body weight (mean of 0.5 kg) compared to weight gain in patients receiving insulin only. Reductions in insulin requirements and body weight are greatest in more obese patients. The optimal timing for administration is immediately before a meal. The recommended starting dose for Type 1 diabetes is 15 μg before each meal, with increases to 60 μg. The recommended initial dose for Type 2 diabetes is 60 μg, titrated upward as tolerated to 120 μg with each meal. Oral medications that require rapid absorption for effectiveness should be administered either 1 hour before or 2 hours after injection of pramlintide. Mild to moderate nausea is the most commonly reported side-effect and generally dissipates by 4 weeks. Nausea can be minimized by slow upward dose titration and is less common in patients with Type 2 diabetes.

GLP-1 therapies

GLP-1 is produced from the proglucagon gene in L-cells of the small intestine and is secreted in response to nutrients. The GLP-1 analogue exenatide is used in the treatment of Type 1 diabetes. GLP-1 exerts its main effect by stimulating glucose-dependent insulin release from the pancreatic islets. It has also been shown to slow gastric emptying, inhibit inappropriate postmeal glucagon release, and reduce food intake. Exenatide is a naturally occurring component of the Gila monster (*Heloderma suspectum*) saliva. It is resistant to dipeptidyl peptidase IV (DPP-IV) degradation and, therefore, exhibits a prolonged half-life. Exenatide is synthetic exendin-4 and is the first GLP-1 based therapy to be approved in the UK for the treatment of Type 2 diabetes in patients not sufficiently controlled with oral agents.

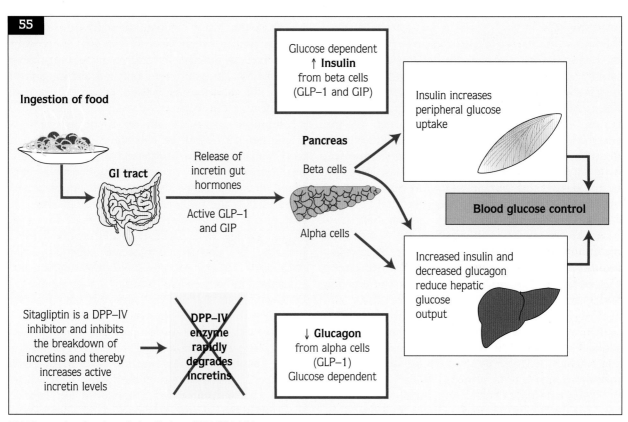

55 The mode of action of sitagliptin, a DPP-IV inhibitor.

Like GLP-1, exenatide exhibits glucose-dependent augmentation of insulin secretion, slows gastric emptying, suppresses inappropriately elevated glucagon levels, and leads to weight loss. Studies of exenatide at a subcutaneous dose of 5–10 µg twice daily, added to sulphonylurea, metformin monotherapy, a combination of sulphonylurea and metformin, or to glitazone therapy show a modest decrease in HbA1c and average weight loss of 1.5–3 kg in the 10 µg group. Exenatide is not currently approved for use with insulin therapy. Nausea is a common adverse effect of exenatide, but is generally mild to moderate in intensity and wanes with duration of therapy. Exenatide is available in prefilled syringes that hold a month's supply of either 5 or 10 µg doses, and is administered subcutaneously twice daily immediately before or within 1 hour of morning and evening meals. Caution is suggested in prescribing for patients with confirmed gastroparesis.

Dipeptidyl peptidase IV (DPP-IV) inhibitors

Dipeptidyl peptidase IV (DPP-IV) is an enzyme that deactivates a variety of other bioactive peptides, including GIP and GLP-1 (55). DPP-IV inhibitors, unlike other GLP-1 based therapies, can be administered orally. Sitagliptin and vildagliptin are DPP-IV inhibitors that are licensed in the UK for treatment of Type 2 diabetes, to be prescribed as either monotherapy or in combination with metformin or a thiazolidinedione. The usual dose of sitagliptin is 100 mg once daily. These drugs result in reductions in HbA1c of 0.4–0.6%, with no difference in body weight or hypoglycaemia. There may be an increased risk of gastrointestinal side-effects. The long-term consequences of DPP-IV inhibition are unknown.

Pramlintide, exenatide and DPP-IV inhibitors reproduce or enhance the actions of naturally occurring peptide hormones and control glucose without causing weight gain. The exact role for these drugs among the myriad of other agents for diabetes management is unclear.

INSULIN THERAPY

Since pancreatic β-cell function deteriorates during the course of Type 2 diabetes, many patients will ultimately require insulin therapy. There will be a variety of emotions encountered at the prospect of this change. Many patients will feel angry, afraid, or guilty. Acceptance of insulin therapy can be made easier if the subject of insulin has been discussed early in the course of the disease. An appropriate educational programme should ensure that this has occurred. Quality of life may be enhanced rather than impaired as a result of insulin therapy being started. Although the addition of insulin can complicate lifestyle, the sense of well being that occurs with resolution of hyperglycaemia can be of greater significance. It is vital during this transitional period that each patient is offered support, encouragement, and appropriate education.

About one-quarter of patients with Type 2 diabetes will require insulin therapy within 10 years of the diagnosis of Type 2 diabetes. It is probable that if glycaemic control is targeted as aggressively as the evidence suggests that it should be, an even greater proportion of patients will require insulin. Insulin may also be required if medical complications ensue or in other specific circumstances. Indications for insulin therapy are presented in *Table 56*.

The insulin regime that is chosen will depend upon the patient's symptoms, the degree of hyperglycaemia, current treatment, coexisting conditions, obesity, and social situation. The decision should be taken in combination with the patient so that individual wishes and sensitivities are taken into account. Commonly used regimes are listed in *Table 57*.

Insulin plus tablets

Regardless of the regime chosen, there is evidence that continuing metformin therapy when insulin is started leads to improved glycaemic control, reduced risk of hyperglycaemia, and less weight gain. It is now standard practice to continue metformin therapy in overweight Type 2 diabetic patients requiring insulin. If daytime glucose control is good but blood glucose levels are high overnight, it may be reasonable to add an overnight dose of a long-acting insulin without discontinuing any oral medication.

Once daily insulin

Commencing once daily insulin therapy as an alternative to tablet treatment may be appropriate for frail elderly patients. This may be the easiest practicable measure to ensure good health when tight blood glucose control is not appropriate. For once daily regimes, the longer-acting insulin analogue Glargine or Determir injected at bedtime may be preferred to a traditional intermediate-acting insulin. NICE currently recommends that Insulin Glargine is

---

Table 56 Indications for insulin therapy

❏ Failure to achieve adequate glycaemic control on maximal oral hypoglycaemic therapy
❏ Failure to tolerate oral hypoglycaemic therapy
❏ Contraindications to oral hypoglycaemic therapy
❏ Weight loss and ketonuria
❏ Acute illness
❏ Perioperative management
❏ Diabetes in pregnancy
❏ Steroid therapy
❏ Severe infection
❏ Acute cardiac ischaemia and myocardial infarction

Table 57 Commonly used insulin regimes in Type 2 diabetes

Regime	Mechanism of introduction
Twice daily	Stop all glucose-lowering therapy except for metformin. Start twice daily intermediate-acting insulin or mixed insulin
Insulin plus tablets	An intermediate-acting or long-acting insulin analogue added at bedtime to tablet therapy
Basal bolus	Commence a rapid-acting insulin before each of three meals, plus an intermediate or long-acting insulin analogue at night (or twice daily). Metformin can be stopped or continued
Once daily	Replacing tablets with a once daily intermediate or long-acting insulin at bedtime (for selected patient types only)

not used routinely for people with Type 2 diabetes who require insulin therapy. However, it should be considered for those who need assistance to administer injections, whose lifestyle is restricted by recurrent hypoglycaemia, or who would otherwise require twice daily injections of insulin in combination with tablet treatment.

Making the change to insulin therapy

Initiating insulin therapy does not generally require inpatient admission. It has traditionally been carried out in a one to one consultation with an appropriately trained health care professional who has the time to address the patient's individual needs and concerns. Traditionally, this has been the diabetes nurse specialist or a diabetes specialist within the hospital setting. This role is now increasingly being extended to those within the primary care setting, e.g. practice nurses. More recently, insulin therapy has been initiated in groups, ideally 6–8 patients. This has the benefit of providing greater peer support in an environment that may be more conducive to learning. The process has the added benefit of being more time-effective. Whichever method is chosen, it is vital that there is easy access to advice, support, and further education once the insulin has been initiated. Ideally, there should be continuity of care provided with the health care professional who initiated insulin therapy.

Insulin is used to improve metabolic control in patients with Type 2 diabetes. It may improve symptoms and should reduce the risk of micro-vascular complications of diabetes. Its use does not come without a price. Weight gain and hypo-glycaemia are the most frequent complications. Weight can increase by an average of 4 kg if insulin is initiated immediately after diet control. The weight gain is less severe when insulin is used to substitute sulphonylurea therapy. Continuation of metformin can help to limit weight gain. Severe hypoglycaemia is less common in Type 2 than in Type 1 diabetes. However, initiating insulin therapy does increase the risk of severe hypoglycaemia. This risk is increased with duration of treatment (see The pathophysiology of Type 2 diabetes and insulin resistance, page 11).

It may be possible to discontinue insulin in patients who have made significant lifestyle changes, particularly when this is associated with weight loss. In addition, some patients started on insulin for a concurrent illness or treatment may subsequently not require insulin therapy. However, patients should only return to tablet therapy or diet alone if there was no suggestion of insulin deficiency (e.g. previous ketosis or low weight). There should be close super-vision if this is attempted.

MANAGING THE CHRONIC COMPLICATIONS OF DIABETES
EYE DISEASE
Treatment of diabetic retinopathy
Laser photocoagulation is the treatment of choice for proliferative retinopathy, worsening preproliferative retinopathy, and maculopathy. The technique can be performed as an outpatient procedure. Local anaesthetic drops are applied to the eye. Using a lens placed on the cornea, an operator sitting at a slit lamp applies the laser. Pan-retinal photocoagulation involves multiple burns (typically about 1500) measuring 500 μm diameter. These are applied in patterns around the temporal blood vessel arcades and to the temporal region of the peripheral retina. This works by reducing the retinal demand for oxygen with a subsequent reduction in vascular endothelium-derived growth factor (VEGF) production that diminishes the stimulus to new vessel formation. Pan-retinal laser photo-coagulation reduces the risk of vitreous haemorrhage and visual loss by 50%. The procedure is usually completed in two or three treatment sessions.

In exudative maculopathy, photocoagulation prevents worsening of maculopathy by reducing oedema and exudative deposit. Circinate rings of hard exudate around the macula benefit from laser therapy applied to the central area of a ring to reduce capillary leakage. This prevents further visual deterioration in more than one-half of subjects.

Cataracts
Surgical treatment is recommended for deteriorating visual loss leading to impaired quality of life. It may also be indicated to allow assessment and treatment of retinopathy to take place. The need for surgery has to be balanced against the possibility that it may worsen retinopathy and maculopathy in those with severe disease, and is also associated with increased morbidity in the perioperative period.

Visual loss due to temporal arteritis
If an erythrocyte sedimentation rate (ESR) is significantly elevated with symptoms of temporal headache, jaw claudication, malaise, and weight loss then high-dose steroids (prednisolone 60 mg) should be started to protect the other eye from the effects of temporal arteritis.

KIDNEY DISEASE
Management of diabetic nephropathy

Any degree of proteinuria is associated with an increased risk of cardiovascular disease. With overt (dipstick-positive) proteinuria, this risk is increased tenfold.

> *In patients with microalbuminuria or overt proteinuria, the aims should be to lower elevated blood pressure, treat cardiovascular risk factors, ensure adequate glucose control, and begin therapy with an ACE inhibitor or angiotensin II receptor antagonist.*

Early effective blood pressure lowering to 140/80 mmHg or below, reduces the rate of decline in glomerular filtration rate (GFR) by more than 50%. Beta-blockers, diuretics, and nondihydropyridine calcium channel blockers (diltiazem, verapamil) are all effective. ACE inhibitor drugs are known, however, to have a greater effect than traditional antihypertensive agents in reducing progression to dialysis and transplantation. They have been widely used and have a good safety profile. ACE inhibitors have also been shown to reduce the progression of microalbuminuria in normotensive patients with Type 1 diabetes. Patients with persistent microalbuminuria should be started on ACE inhibitor therapy titrated to moderate/high dose to obtain maximum benefit. Along with angiotensin II blockers, the ACE inhibitor class of drugs has been shown to have similar benefits in patients with Type 2 diabetes. (Angiotensin II blockers are frequently prescribed when ACE inhibitors cannot be used due to side-effects [typically, a dry cough].)

Patients commencing these agents should have blood taken for urea and electrolytes before and within 1 week after commencing therapy. This is to ensure there is no deterioration in renal function due to underlying renal artery stenosis, since both ACE inhibitors and angiotensin II blockers exacerbate this condition. Although good glucose control is a major factor in determining the progression to micro-albuminuria, the risk improves very significantly once HbA1c exceeds 8.1%. Although it is not known whether this benefit extends to those with established microalbuminuria, there will undoubtedly be benefits for other microvascular complications such as retinopathy. Aggressive treatment of cardiovascular risk factors such as hyperlipidaemia and smoking is essential in diabetic patients with proteinuria.

Nephrotic syndrome

This is a less common manifestation of diabetic nephropathy. The prognosis is poor since the condition is associated with rapidly progressive renal failure. Nephrotic range proteinuria leads to hypoalbuminaemia and peripheral oedema. The key to management is control of fluid balance and blood pressure. Diuresis needs to be optimized to avoid dehydration and worsening renal function. ACE inhibitor therapy should form part of the antihypertensive regime. A high protein diet is recommended to help maintain serum protein levels.

Examination of the urine microscopically should be carried out. The presence of red cells and casts suggests an alternative diagnosis, such as glomerulonephritis, and a renal biopsy should be performed.

Renal failure

Progressive renal failure is accompanied by hypertension and fluid retention. Management takes the following course:

❑ A blood pressure of 135/75 mmHg should be targeted but may not be obtainable despite several antihypertensive agents.

❑ Fluid retention is controlled with loop diuretics although a thiazide diuretic may also need to be added.

❑ Excessive protein and salt intake should be avoided, but severe dietary protein restriction to delay worsening of renal function is now rarely advocated.

As worsening renal failure develops, treatment regimes need to be re-assessed. Metformin should be stopped at serum creatinine levels of >150 µmol/l due to the increased risk of lactic acidosis. Sulphonylureas are renally excreted and it is important to avoid long-acting sulphonylurea drugs in patients with renal failure.

In Type 2 diabetes, the limitations of oral therapy frequently result in a switch to insulin therapy. Insulin, however, is cleared renally and the dose of insulin used in diabetes may need to be reduced by as much as half in established renal failure. Careful blood glucose and HbA1c monitoring are required as renal function deteriorates.

> *Referral to a specialist renal department should be considered once the creatinine is above 150 µmol/l.*
> *With levels >500 µmol/l, the patient should be considered for renal transplantation.*

Older patients (aged >65 years) have a high risk of cardiovascular disease and a poor prognosis. These patients may be offered dialysis rather than transplantation once they require renal replacement therapy. Those who are waiting for, or are inappropriate for, transplantation are offered dialysis therapy. Unlike haemodialysis, chronic ambulatory peritoneal dialysis (CAPD) does not require vascular access. This is particularly useful in diabetes, since vascular access may be technically difficult due to atherosclerosis and vessel wall calcification that can lead to failure of arterio-venous fistulae. CAPD is also more suitable for elderly patients, those with cardiac failure, and autonomic neuropathy. This is because extracellular fluid volumes and blood pressure are stable.

CAPD has the additional advantage that insulin can be administered into the peritoneal cavity during treatment. This helps to stabilize blood glucose concentration.

Renal transplantation may be cadaveric or occasionally from a living related donor. Although patient and graft survival rates are slightly inferior to those of nondiabetic patients, the presence of diabetes should not prevent the opportunity of transplantation for those with diabetes. The patient survival rate is >80% at 5 years for those receiving grafts from living related donors. All those being considered for transplantation should have coronary investigations to assess cardiovascular risk.

Renal artery stenosis (RAS)

RAS may be treated by percutaneous angioplasty (PTCA) to improve renal blood supply. Results, however, in those with diabetes are not as good as those in nondiabetic individuals.

NEUROPATHY AND FOOT DISEASE

Management of diabetic neuropathy (sensorimotor neuropathy and neuropathic pain)

It has now been shown that the risk of developing neuropathy can be significantly reduced with tight blood glucose control in both Type 1 and Type 2 diabetes. Patients with sensorimotor neuropathy should be identified as having a high risk for the development of diabetic foot ulceration. Screening for neuropathy enables appropriate footwear and foot care advice to be directed towards these sufferers.

There is a variety of treatments available for the management of neuropathic pain, but success in alleviating all pain may be unrealistic for many. The goal of treatment is an improved quality of life, improved sleep, and a reduction in pain. The response to differing treatments will vary markedly between individuals. Improvement in glycaemic control may help prevent the development and progression of neuropathic pain. It is important to target a lowering of blood glucose in those patients who have poor control, but painful neuropathic symptoms can worsen acutely in the context of sudden deterioration or improvement in glycaemic control. The aim should, therefore, be a gradual improvement. Patients with Type 2 diabetes and poor glucose control despite maximal oral hypoglycaemic agents should be commenced on insulin therapy.

Neuropathic pain is usually a self-limiting condition, but symptoms can last for many years. It is important to inform sufferers about the cause and natural history of this condition. This information should include a careful explanation of different treatments, their effectiveness, potential side-effects, and likely improvements. It is essential that quick access for contact and support is available. It is common for patients to require a number of different treatments, either alone or in combination. Treatment should be monitored and adjusted in order to maximize the beneficial effects. This may be achieved more easily by involving patients in their management through self-titration of drug therapy and agreed care protocols.

Simple painkillers such as paracetamol are rarely effective for neuropathic pain and their use should not be prolonged unless there is a rapid response to treatment. Topical agents include capsaicin cream derived from the chilli pepper. This is applied three to four times daily to symptomatic areas of the foot. It is believed to work through depletion of substance P from nerve terminals. Capsaicin cream should be reserved for superficial discomfort and pain (burning, tingling). Symptoms may worsen for a period of 2–4 weeks following its initial use, and the full benefit may not be realized for 6 weeks. It is essential that patients are well educated in the use of this product in order for it to be effective. Hands need to be washed before and immediately after use. Contact with eyes and inflamed or broken skin should be avoided. It should not be used under tight bandages. The patient should also avoid taking a hot shower or bath immediately before or after applying the cream since this exacerbates the burning sensation.

'Opsite' spray is an alternative topical therapy that is sprayed directly onto the affected area and can give dramatic relief. This treatment can unfortunately be somewhat messy, leaving behind a filmy residue. Tricyclic antidepressant medication has, for many years, been a first-line systemic therapy effective in neuropathic pain. Imipramine and amitryptiline have been shown to be beneficial in up to 60% of symptomatic patients. Doses should be started low (25–50 mg) and titrated upwards slowly. Side-effects include sedation, dry mouth, urinary retention, postural hypotension, and exacerbation of glaucoma.

The anticonvulsants gabapentin (Neurontin) and its more recent successor pregabalin (Lyrica) are licensed as oral agents for use in painful neuropathy. Common side-effects are dizziness and drowsiness. Pregabalin may have benefits over its predecessor. Dose titration is simpler and quicker. Benefits are seen within 1 week of therapy and improvements in sleep pattern changes are noticeable. The usual final treatment dose is 150–300 mg twice daily. Carbamazepine and phenytoin have been used in the treatment of neuropathic pain, but side-effects are common and these drugs are now used less frequently. Opiate-based therapies can cause dependence, but may be advocated in severe intractable cases. Tramadol is a centrally acting opioid derivative that is less addictive and has been shown to benefit some patients with neuropathic pain. A typical daily dose is 200–400 mg.

Other more invasive but occasionally successful therapies have included intravenous lignocaine, intramuscular ketamine, spinal cord stimulation with transcutaneous electrical nerve stimulation (TENS) machines, and spinal nerve blocks. These should only be considered within specialist settings. Complementary and physical therapies can be used as an adjunct to conventional therapies. For some individuals they can be useful in reducing the impact of this painful condition on quality of life and daily function. These include relaxation and mind body techniques, herbal remedies, therapeutic massage, chiropractice, reflexology, acupuncture, and magnetic therapy.

Diabetic amyotrophy
The pain associated with this condition may respond to tricyclic agents. The primary aim of treatment, however, is to improve glucose control.

Entrapment neuroathies such as carpal tunnel syndrome
Definitive treatment is by surgical decompression although surgical splints and analgesia may be effective management for some.

Autonomic neuropathy
Postural hypotension can be eased by avoiding dehydration, assuming a standing position more slowly, support stockings to speed venous return, and lifting the head of the bed overnight. Drugs likely to exacerbate the problem should be avoided where possible. Fludrocortisone therapy at doses up to 0.4 mg daily can be very helpful. Mitodrine, desmopressin, and somatostatin analogues have also been used cautiously with some success.

Abnormal sweating can be helped by propantheline bromide, typically 15 mg three times daily and 30 mg at night. Diabetic gastroparesis is a difficult condition to manage. Metoclopramide, cisapride, and domperidone can be effective for vomiting. Anti-diarrhoeal agents and a short course of oral tetracycline may help symptoms of diarrhoea. Symptoms of gastroparesis are typically worse during periods of infection or ill health. Hospital admission to control blood glucose levels may occasionally be required.

Managing the ischaemic foot
Patients with ischaemic ulceration or rest pain should receive consideration for further investigation with a view to surgical therapy. In view of the increased cardiovascular risk, this is assessed on an individual basis. The increased emphasis on limb salvage and the development of new techniques of re-vascularization has led to a reduction in the frequency of major amputation in patients with diabetic foot ulceration. The conventional noninvasive technique for identifying limb ischaemia is Doppler ultrasound. This assesses the velocity of blood flow and the pressure index within lower limb arteries. It can, however, be unreliable in patients with significant arterial wall calcification. Combination with duplex ultrasound demonstrates the anatomy and function of vessels in more detail. Digital subtraction arteriography has enabled better views of diseased distal limb vessels prior to interventional treatment.

Angioplasty has now become established in the treatment of diabetic peripheral vascular disease. Modern catheters use balloons to dilate strictures. Arterial bypass therapy in diabetes is difficult because of the distal and diffuse nature of the atherosclerotic disease. However, in carefully selected patients, limb salvage and graft patency are improved in distal bypass grafts to both the dorsalis pedis and posterior tibial arteries. The re-vascularization of feet via distal arterial reconstruction appears to provide good capillary perfusion despite the presence of diabetes.

Although this form of surgery may require repeat surgical procedures, the cost is less than that of major amputation. The use of autologous vein grafts rather than prosthetic grafts has further increased patency and limb salvage rates.

Managing diabetic foot ulceration

In the initial stages of acute foot ulceration it is important to reduce weight-bearing. This is essential to promote healing. Bed rest is not generally advised since prolonged immobilization should be avoided as it may lead to thrombo-embolic and other complications. Care should be taken to prevent pressure on the heels with pressure-relieving boots and mattresses. Casting techniques offer an alternative to bed rest since they allow the patient to retain mobility. These include total contact plaster cast with simple padding, removable casts such as the Scotch cast boot, and removable cast walkers such as the Aircast pneumatic diabetic walking boot.

Pressure can also be reduced with moulded polyethylene foam insoles. When using moulded insoles it is important that shoes have more depth, uppers should be flexible, heels should be stable, and the forefoot area of the shoe wide and square. Lace-ups prevent foot slippage and resultant trauma to the end of toes. Shoes need to be customized individually (bespoke) where foot deformity is present. For an ulcer situated beneath a metatarsal head, a common adjustment includes a metatarsal bar that is placed proximal to the metatarsal heads. A rocker sole can be useful for ulcers beneath the first toe since it shifts the pressure load to the mid-foot.

A foot ulcer is surrounded by callus and this needs to be surgically removed. This has the effect of reducing local pressure, allowing effective drainage of the wound, enabling re-epithelialization of the ulcer edges. It should result in an improved rate of healing. The blade of a scalpel is used to pare away the callus so that the base of the ulcer is fully exposed. The wound and the surrounding skin should then be cleaned with a sterile saline solution. The ulcer should be covered with a clean nonadhesive dressing. This procedure will frequently need to be repeated until the ulcer is healed.

There is evidence that growth factor-containing gels and membranes may improve the healing rate of diabetic foot ulceration, but the cost may be prohibitive and their use may be restricted to difficult nonhealing ulcers.

For infected ulcers, high-dose, broad-spectrum antibiotic therapy is advocated. Tissue penetration may be poor and low doses of antibiotic may lead to inadequate levels within the target tissue. Coamoxiclav in the form of 'Augmentin' 625 mg three times daily for a period of 2 weeks is a recommended treatment regime. In the presence of spreading cellulitis, surrounding erythema, or skin discolouration, the use of intravenous antibiotics is indicated. A combination of cefuroxime and metronidazole is common, but will depend upon whether there is bone involvement and whether there is an increased risk of methicillin resistant *Staphylococcus aureus* (MRSA). In this case, intravenous vancomycin may be added.

Collections of pus and abscess cavities need surgical drainage. Necrotic tissue should be removed surgically. Gangrene in a digit requires a ray amputation, i.e. the surgical removal of the affected phalanx and metatarsal head.

Managing the Charcot foot

The key to treatment is immobilization. This will prevent further joint damage and should be recommended immediately. Continued walking will inevitably lead to ulceration and more damage. Options include crutches, wheelchair, total contact cast, and a replaceable cast walker. These allow patients to mobilize safely and usually without pain. Immobilization is recommended for a period of 2–3 months but can be as long as 1 year depending upon the activity of the disease.

Bisphosphonates such as pamidronate may be administered by intravenous infusion. These can reduce swelling, pain, and redness and work by reducing osteoclast activity. When the acute phase has resolved, the foot should be reviewed and future care must be planned. The patient should be considered at high risk for ulceration and appropriate footwear and follow-up assessment should be arranged. An orthopaedic opinion for consideration of reconstructive surgery may be useful in helping to restore normal foot shape.

ERECTILE DYSFUNCTION (ED)

Before initiating drug therapy for ED, the following considerations should be addressed:

❏ Endocrine causes for ED need to be identified and treated.

❏ Offending drugs should be withdrawn where this is safe and reasonable.

❏ Smoking cessation should be advised and glucose control optimized.

❏ Simple psychological concerns should be addressed.

❑ Significant psychological or psychiatric problems require specialist psychosexual input.

Sildenafil (Viagra) was the first oral treatment for ED. It selectively inhibits phosphodiesterase-5 (PD-5), an enzyme that breaks down intracellular cyclic guanosine monophosphate (GMP). This causes smooth muscle relaxation and improves penile blood flow. It is effective in the presence of sexual stimulation but does not cause spontaneous erections or increase libido. Subsequently, the other PD-5 inhibitors, vardenafil and tadalafil, have been introduced. These have a slightly quicker onset of action (about 30 rather than 60 minutes). Tadalafil has a longer duration of action than the others (36 hours).

These drugs are contraindicated in patients with hypotension, recent stroke or MI, severe hepatic impairment, or hereditary degenerative retinal disorders. They should not be coprescribed with oral nitrates, nicorandil, and some antiviral agents. Side-effects of this group of drugs include headache, flushing and, in the case of sildenafil, bluish-green visual disturbance. These drugs are available on prescription for those with diabetes. Only one tablet per week can be prescribed on the National Health Service, although they can be taken once daily. The lowest dose should be started and increased gradually if ineffective. The tablet is taken prior to planned sexual activity. These treatments are effective in around two-thirds of patients.

Apomorphine (uprima) is an alternative noninvasive therapy for ED. It is a sublingual preparation that acts centrally on neuronal transmitters in the hypothalamus. It leads to secondary relaxation of smooth muscle in the corpus cavernosum via oxytocinergic pathways. It can be given within 20 minutes of intercourse at a dose of 2–3 mg. Alternative treatments include transurethral alprostadil (MUSE), intracavernosal alprostadil injections (caverject and viridal), vacuum devices, and penile prostheses. These treatments used to be the mainstay of ED management but are now rarely used other than in cases of tablet failure. Intraurethral alprostadil (prostaglandin E1) is in the form of a soluble tablet inserted directly into the urethra with an applicator. Self-administration should only take place after proper training. It should not be used more than seven times during the course of a week. If a partner is fertile then appropriate barrier contraception should be used.

Intracorporeal injection therapy is an alternative self-administered technique that was the most popular method of treating ED until recent years. After an initial training period, patients can adjust dose requirements according to response. This should not be given more than three times weekly. Complications include penile pain, priapism, and penile fibrosis.

Vacuum tumescence devices are safe and effective but are somewhat clumsy and obtrusive. These devices mostly work on a similar principle. A cylinder is placed over the penis and a connecting pump used to pump air out to create a vacuum. This leads to a tumescent penis. Over the base of the erect penis a rubber ring is placed to maintain the erection. This technique allows an erection sufficient for intercourse in over 80% of patients. They can cause bruising and discomfort and do need to be funded by the patient. Penile prostheses are used for patients who have failed to respond to other therapies. They can be permanent, mechanical, or inflatable. Complications are common and include infection, mechanical failure, pain, and bruising. A management algorithm of ED is presented in figure 56.

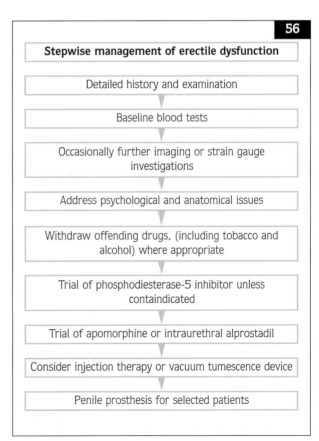

56

Stepwise management of erectile dysfunction

Detailed history and examination

Baseline blood tests

Occasionally further imaging or strain gauge investigations

Address psychological and anatomical issues

Withdraw offending drugs, (including tobacco and alcohol) where appropriate

Trial of phosphodiesterase-5 inhibitor unless containdicated

Trial of apomorphine or intraurethral alprostadil

Consider injection therapy or vacuum tumescence device

Penile prosthesis for selected patients

56 Algorithm for the management of erectile dysfunction.

CASE 3

A 35-year-old man with a 20-year history of Type 1 diabetes is having a routine eye inspection. He is symptom free. The following left fundus (57) is visualized.

1 What is the diagnosis?
2 What should be done and how quickly?

Answers to Case 3 on page 157.

57 Case 3: left fundus.

MANAGING DIABETES IN PREGNANCY

Optimal blood glucose control is essential to reduce the risks of fetal complications. Most patients will require a basal bolus system of insulin administration. Instruction on how to adjust diet, lifestyle, and insulin dose to obtain tight glucose control is essential. Frequent blood glucose monitoring is required and target blood glucose levels should be <5 mmol/l preprandially and <7 mmol/l postprandially. Although not licensed in pregnancy, some centres are using quick-acting insulin analogues to help achieve good control. Insulin pump therapy is an alternative management strategy, particularly for those who suffer with severe recurrent hypoglycaemia. Frequent (monthly) HbA1c or fructosamine measurements are required to confirm home readings.

Insulin requirements tend to increase gradually in the second trimester until about 36 weeks gestation.

> *Glucagon should be offered to women who are at risk of severe hypoglycaemia. Training should be given to the partner or person most likely to administer it.*

Screening for complications is essential during pregnancy. Retinal screening should be carried out regularly. Established retinopathy, particularly proliferative and preproliferative disease, may worsen dramatically during pregnancy. Occasionally, prophylactic laser therapy is required. Pregnancy can worsen established renal failure. Blood pressure should be tightly controlled in this situation. A combination of nifedipine and/or methyldopa is commonly used. Regular obstetric assessment in combination with a diabetes assessment is essential in order to recognize and manage complications. Regular ultrasound scans are required to assess fetal age, growth, malformations, and the presence of polyhydramnios.

MANAGING DIABETES DURING AND AFTER DELIVERY

During labour, blood glucose is managed with an insulin infusion combined with a dextrose and potassium infusion. Local guidelines should be followed. This frequently employs a sliding scale regimen with hourly blood glucose monitoring. During labour women are able to detect hypoglycaemia and it is therefore reasonable to aim for blood glucose levels of 4–8 mmol/l. This reduces the risk of fetal hypoglycaemia occurring as a result of glucose crossing the placenta from maternal circulation and stimulating fetal insulin production.

After delivery of the placenta, mothers with Type 1 diabetes should return to insulin doses that were used in the first trimester. Those with gestational diabetes who have been commenced on insulin during pregnancy can cease insulin. Mothers with Type 1 diabetes who decide to breast feed are likely to require a reduction of insulin dose (about 10%) in addition to taking regular snacks.

ENDOCRINOLOGY

MANAGING THYROID DISEASE
THYROTOXICOSIS

There are three forms of treatment available for the management of thyrotoxicosis: drug therapy, radioiodine, and surgery.

Drug therapy

Antithyroid drug therapy is frequently recommended as first-line therapy in Graves' disease. Carbimazole is often the drug of choice in the UK since it can be given as a once daily preparation. During pregnancy and breast feeding, propylthiouracil is often given instead since it is not associated with fetal abnormalities and has a lower concentration in breast milk. Propylthiouracil has a quicker onset of action than carbimazole since, in addition to preventing the uptake of iodine into the thyroid gland, it also inhibits the conversion of free T4 to free T3. The most common side-effects are gastrointestinal (nausea and dyspepsia). Allergic reactions (rash and arthralgia) occur in a small percentage of patients but frequently settle spontaneously.

The most severe side-effect is agranulocytosis; this occurs in less than 1 in 200 patients and is most frequent in the first 3 months of administration. Patients should be instructed to stop the drug and have a full blood count measured should they develop a fever, sore throat, or become unwell.

Antithyroid drugs can be dose titrated or given as a block and replace regimen in combination with thyroxine. The usual starting dose of carbimazole is 30–40 mg daily. This can be titrated every 6 weeks. The final dose is usually 5–10 mg. The aim should be to obtain a seum thyroid stimulating hormone (TSH) level that lies within the normal range on blood testing. Propylthiouracil is started at a dose of 300–400 mg in 2–3 divided doses daily, and is titrated down to a maintenace of 50–150 mg in most patients. If a block and replace regime is used, a dose of thyroxine (starting at 100 µg) is added to 40 mg carbimazole as soon as the patient is euthyroid.

If adequately drug treated for 12–18 months, 60% of patients will have a relapse within 10 years.

Radioiodine therapy

Radioiodine is a common alternative to continuing drug treatment. This treatment consists of iodine-131 is given as a capsule or a drink at a dose of 400–800 MBq. This dose gives a cure rate of 90%.

Radioiodine usually takes effect within 6–8 weeks of administration. Patients are asked to discontinue antithyroid drugs 2–5 days prior to administration and can recommence 3 days after treatment. If required, a second dose should be given 6 months after the first.

Half of all treated patients with Graves' disease are rendered hypothyroid within 10 years, the majority within the first few months of treatment. These patients will usually require permanent thyroxine replacement although early postradio-iodine hypothyroidism may be transient. The incidence of hypothyroidism after radioiodine therapy in patients with thyrotoxicosis caused by a hot nodule(s) is less common.

Patients receiving radioiodine should be instructed to avoid close contact with others, particularly children, for 2 weeks and should avoid pregnancy for 4 months following treatment. *Table 58* presents the indications and contraindications for radioiodine therapy.

Table 58 Indications and contraindications for radioiodine therapy

Indications
- ❑ Relapsed Graves' disease following a course of drug therapy
- ❑ Patients with a high risk of relapse on drug therapy (young age, large goitres, extrathyroid manifestations of Graves' disease, strongly-positive antibodies, large doses of antithyroid drugs)
- ❑ Single toxic nodule
- ❑ Toxic multinodular goitre
- ❑ Drug intolerance
- ❑ Patient preference

Contraindications
- ❑ Severe Graves' ophthalmopathy
- ❑ Children (<14 years)
- ❑ Pregnancy or breast feeding
- ❑ Risks to others (e.g. close contact to child required)

Graves' ophthalmopathy may worsen after the administration of radioiodine. If radioiodine is given then high doses of prednisolone (40 mg tailed off over 2 months) should be prescribed. This may prevent a relapse of the eye disease. Amiodarone and other iodine containing products (including some vitamin and mineral supplements) block the uptake of iodine by the thyroid gland and render radioiodine ineffective. The prolonged half-life of amiodarone means that radioiodine is ineffective for many months after the drug is discontinued.

Surgery

Surgery is now rarely the treatment of choice in uncomplicated Graves' disease. However, there are a number of situations in which its use should be considered:

❏ Malignant or suspicious thyroid nodule.
❏ Pregnancy where drug treatment is ineffective (second trimester).
❏ Poor compliance or poor control with drug therapy.
❏ Local compressive symptoms.
❏ Severe Graves' ophthalmopathy.
❏ Large goitre.
❏ Patient preference.

Patients should be prepared for surgery with drug therapy to render them euthyroid (normal thyroid function) before any operation is considered. Potassium iodide 60 mg t.d.s. for 10 days may reduce the vascularity of the thyroid gland. In patients with uncontrolled thyrotoxicosis, steroid therapy and beta-blockers may also be used prior to surgery if the euthyroid state cannot be achieved and surgery is considered essential. Subtotal thyroidectomy is the most commonly performed procedure. The rate of subsequent hypothyroidism (10–50%) depends upon the size of thyroid remnant left behind. *Table 59* lists the potential complications of surgery.

Graves' disease-associated complications

The treatment of Graves' ophthalmopathy is frequently symptomatic with artificial tears or the taping of eyes at night to reduce corneal abrasion. In more severe cases, systemic steroids, immunosuppressant drugs (e.g. azathioprine) and radiotherapy may be required. Occasionally, surgical orbit decompression or eye muscle surgery is required.

Treatment of pretibial myxoedema is reserved for severe cases. Potent topical and systemic steroids can cause some resolution of pain and tenderness. There is

---

Table 59 Complications of thyroid surgery

Early
❏ Haemorrhage
❏ Infection
❏ Hypoparathyroidism
❏ Damage to recurrent laryngeal nerve
❏ Thyroid crisis (rare)

Late
❏ Hypothyroidism
❏ Recurrent thyrotoxicosis (rare)
❏ Scar formation

---

no treatment available for thyroid acropachy but it is usually painless.

Subacute infective (De Quervain's) thyroiditis

This self-limiting condition can be managed with nonsteroidal anti-inflammatory drug (NSAID) therapy with propanolol to control symptoms. In more severe cases, prednisolone 30 mg daily is effective. Carbimazole and propylthiouracil should be avoided since they will render the patient hypothyroid.

Secondary hyperthyroidism

The treatment of pituitary-dependent hyperthyroidism is surgical removal of the TSH secreting adenoma. Other treatment options include pituitary irradiation and somatostatin analogue therapy.

Management of thyroid disease in pregnancy

Patients should be counselled to avoid pregnancy while being actively managed for thyrotoxicosis or if within 4 months of receiving radioiodine therapy. Key management points include:

❏ Block and replace regimes should be avoided.
❏ Propylthiouracil is the drug of choice since there is less placental transfer.
❏ Radioiodine should not be given.
❏ Breast-feeding mothers should be treated with propylthiouracil at low doses.
❏ T4 should be measured monthly.
❏ Circulating TSH receptor antibodies should be measured at the beginning of the third trimester.

❏ Where antibodies are positive, a fetal heart rate above 160 bpm suggests fetal thyrotoxicosis and the dose of antithyroid drug should be increased.

❏ If increased drug doses render the mother hypothyroid, T4 should be prescribed.

Postpartum thyrotoxicosis

This condition presents in the first 3 months postpartum and there may be secondary lymphocytic infiltration and destruction of the gland. It is managed with beta-blockers since the thyrotoxic phase is typically followed by hypothyroidism beginning 3–6 months postpartum. A ^{99}technetium uptake scan will differentiate between this (reduced uptake) and Graves' disease (increased uptake).

Thyroid crisis

This acute life threatening manifestation of thyrotoxicosis requires prompt therapy. It frequently presents with tachycardia or a tachyarrhythmia and is associated with fever, dehydration, circulatory collapse, and multi-organ failure. If suspected, treatment should be initiated before thyroid function test results become available. *Table 60* presents important management steps in thyroid crisis.

Table 60 Important management steps in thyroid crisis

❏ Patient is best managed in a high dependency setting
❏ Circulatory, cardiovascular, and thermoregulatory dysfunction should be corrected
❏ Electrolyte abnormalities should be corrected
❏ Patients should be screened and treated for systemic infection if suspected
❏ Antiarrhythmic drugs can be used but amiodarone should be avoided
❏ Propylthiouracil 200 mg q.d.s. (via naso-gastric [n-g] tube if necessary)
❏ Potassium iodide 60 mg q.d.s. via n-g
❏ Propranolol 80 mg t.d.s. via n-g or 3 mg/h IV
❏ Prednisolone 60 mg daily via n-g or 50 mg q.d.s. IV
❏ Plasmapheresis can be tried in resistant cases

HYPOTHYROIDISM

Chronic hypothyroidism

Patients with an underactive thyroid gland should be commenced on thyroxine. The starting dose is 50–100 µg once daily. In older patients or in those with ischaemic heart disease or cardiac dysrhythmias, the starting dose should be reduced to 25 µg. The dose should be increased by increments of 50 µg (or 25 µg in high risk individuals) every 4–6 weeks according to levels of free T4. The TSH levels return to normal more slowly but once the patient is stabilized on treatment the aim should be to normalize TSH levels.

Optimal thyroid replacement

Residual symptoms, particularly tiredness, are common following correction of thyroid dysfunction. The mechanisms are unclear. The aim of therapy should be to keep patients symptom free with a free T4 in the upper end of the normal range and a TSH concentration that is within the normal range. The use of free T3 and nonsynthetic thyroid hormone replacement to treat hypothyroidism is controversial. There is evidence that supplementation of T4 with small doses of T3 (in the form of liothyronine sodium) may relieve symptoms in a minority of patients.

The usual therapeutic dose of thyroxine is 100–150 µg daily. However, there is significant variation between individuals and the dose range is 25-200 µg daily.

Once stabilized, thyroid function tests, particularly TSH, should be checked on an annual basis. If large doses of thyroxine are failing to correct hypothyroidism then lack of compliance with medication should be considered.

Management of acute severe hypothyroidism (myxoedema coma)

Hypothyroidism can present acutely, typically with hypothermia. The mortality rate is high. The patient should be rewarmed slowly. Blood pressure, oxygen saturation, urine output, and central venous pressure (CVP) should be monitored and managed appropriately. Glucose and electrolyte abnormalities should be corrected. Concurrent illnesses or infection should be identified and treated. Blood should be taken for thyroid function, cortisol, glucose, full blood count, creatinine, and electrolytes. If there is a suspicion of cortisol deficiency, hydrocortisone 100 mg t.d.s. should be administered intravenously prior to giving thyoxine replacement. Thyroxine should be given at a dose of

300 µg intravenously or via a nasogastric tube immediately. This should be followed by a further 100 µg dose daily. If there is no early improvement, T3 can be added intravenously (25 µg given 8 hourly).

THYROID LUMPS

Thyroid nodules and multinodular goitre

Any overactivity of the thyroid gland should first be corrected with antithyroid drugs, e.g. carbimazole. Once the patient is euthyroid, radioiodine is the first-line therapy for a toxic nodule or toxic multinodular goitre. Surgery is generally reserved for three clinical situations:

❑ Suspicion of malignancy.
❑ Cosmetic disfigurement.
❑ Compression on adjacent structure causing symptoms.

Surgical therapy consists of total or subtotal thyroidectomy. Total thyroidectomy is always recommended for malignancy and will leave patients requiring thyroxine replacement. Following a subtotal thyroidectomy, thyroid function should be checked at 1 month to ascertain whether long-term thyroxine replacement is necessary.

CASE 4

A 24-year-old woman presents to her General Practitioner. She is complaining of anxiety, weight loss (8 kg over a 2 month period) and palpitations. On examination she has a tachycardia (pulse rate 122 bpm) with a fine tremor. Eye examination reveals bilateral proptosis with a full range of eye movements and no diplopia. She has brisk reflexes. She has a smooth diffusely-enlarged goitre palpable in her neck. Thyroid function blood tests are ordered and the results are shown.

Results (normal range)
Free T4 31.3 pmol/l (10.3–24.5)
Thyroid stimulating hormone (TSH) <0.01 nmol/l (0.4–4.0)

1 What is the diagnosis?
2 What medical treatments should be initiated?

CASE 5

A 67-year-old woman presents in the Outpatient Clinic with a history of tiredness and weight gain. She also complains of reduced concentration abilities, increasing hair loss from her scalp, and 'feeling cold all the time'. Her past medical history includes moderate heart failure and ongoing symptomatic angina. On examination she has central obesity, her voice is hoarse, her pulse rate is slow (58 bpm), and her scalp and eyebrow hair is thin. Thyroid function tests are carried out and the results are shown.

Results (normal range)
Free T4 6.8 pmol/l (10.3–24.5)
Thyroid stimulating hormone (TSH) 68 nmol/l (0.4–4.0)

1 What is the diagnosis?
2 What treatment should be initiated and at what dose?

Answers to Cases 4 & 5 on page 157.

MANAGING PARATHYROID DISEASE
HYPERCALCAEMIA AND HYPERPARATHYROIDISM

Hypercalcaemia frequently leads to dehydration. Patients with very high serum calcium levels (>3.5 mmol/l) are usually fluid depleted and may require 3–6 litres of normal saline over a 24 hour period to rehydrate adequately. The intravenous fluids act as a volume expander and increases the GFR, thereby promoting calcium excretion.

The rate of hydration should be determined by the severity of the hypercalcaemia, extent of dehydration, and the patient's cardiovascular reserve.

Once the patient is euvolaemic, a loop diuretic can be given (e.g. 20–40 mg of intravenous frusemide, every 2–12 hours). Bisphosphonates are used once adequate hydration is achieved and if the patient remains hypercalcaemic (>3 mmol/l). They inhibit bone turnover by reducing osteoclastic activity. They are relatively nontoxic, the main side-effects being fever, nausea, and hypomagnesaemia. They tend to be ineffective in hyperparathyroidism.

The newer generation of bisphosphonates are very effective at reducing the calcium concentration quickly. Their maximal effect is seen after 2–4 days. The main intravenous bisphosphonates used in the UK are pamidronate and clodronate.

Clodronate is given intravenously over 4–5 consecutive days (300 mg/day). It can also be given orally (800–1600 mg b.d.) once normocalcaemia is achieved. Pamidronate reduces the calcium concentration more dramatically than clodronate. It is given as a single intravenous infusion of 30–90 mg over 1–2 hours. It is generally well tolerated, but can cause drug fevers. Its effect can last 2–4 weeks. Repeated doses can be given after 7 days.

Calcitonin is a 32-aminoacid polypeptide produced by the parafollicular cells of the thyroid gland, which inhibits osteoclast activity and reduces renal calcium resorption. Calcitonin is administered intramuscularly or subcutaneously. It is safe and reduces calcium quickly (2–6 hours); however, the reduction in calcium is small (approximately 0.5 mmol/l). Glucocorticoids are mainly reserved for patients with chronic granulomatous disorders (e.g. sarcoid) or in patients with vitamin D intoxication. Prednisolone (40–60 mg daily) will usually take 2–5 days to work.

Primary hyperparathyroidism

The only effective proven treatment for primary hyperparathyroidism is surgical removal of the diseased gland(s). Surgery should be considered if any of the following criteria are met:

- ❏ Serum total calcium >3 mmol/l.
- ❏ Episode of life threatening hypercalcaemia.
- ❏ Reduced creatinine clearance.
- ❏ Elevated 24-hour urinary calcium concentration.
- ❏ Nephrolithiasis.
- ❏ Reduced bone mass.
- ❏ Neuromuscular symptoms, e.g. proximal myopathy and gait disturbance.
- ❏ Age <50 years old.

There are three possible types of operation, subtotal parathyroidectomy, total parathyroidectomy, and total parathyroidectomy with autotransplantation.

In subtotal parathyroidectomy, the abnormal tissue is removed, leaving some normal parathyroid tissue behind. This frequently involves the removal of just one affected gland. All the parathyroid tissue is removed in total parathyroidectomy. In total parathyroidectomy and autotransplantation, total parathyroidectomy is accompanied by the implantation of normal parathyroid tissue dissected from the patient's own glands into the patient's forearm. This implant acts as functioning parathyroid tissue.

The advent of high quality scanning demonstrating some 80% of parathyroids has resulted in parathyroid surgeons exploring only one area of the neck if the parathyroid tumour is seen on Sestamibi scanning. The identification of affected parathyroid glands can be aided by injection of methylene blue into the arterial supply at operation. Uncertainty over whether all affected parathyroid glands have been removed can be helped by immediate intraoperative frozen section analysis of removed parathyroid tissue, and by intraoperative parathyroid hormone measurement.

The production of antibodies to parathyroid hormone related protein (PTHrP) has shown initial success by reducing hypercalcaemia and may provide an effective alternative therapy.

Secondary hyperparathyroidism

Targeting the underlying cause of the hypocalcaemia driving the excess parathyroid hormone (PTH) secretion treats secondary hyperparathyroidism and replaces calcium and vitamin D for patients deficient in these.

Tertiary hyperparathyroidism

When there is evidence that the glands are becoming autonomous and hypercalcaemia occurs, total parathyroidectomy should be peformed. The exact type of operation performed depends on each individual situation. The main operation performed in this case is total parathyroidectomy followed by vitamin D and calcium supplementation.

HYPOCALCAEMIA AND HYPOPARATHYROIDISM

Patients suffering with seizures or painful tetany secondary to hypocalcaemia need urgent therapy. *Table 61* outlines the acute management of hypocalcaemia. In hypoparathyroidism and pseudohypoparathyroidism, pharmacological doses of vitamin D such as 0.5–1 µg daily of alphacalcidol are usually required to restore serum calcium levels to the bottom end of the serum calcium reference range. Restoring serum calcium to normal or high normal levels increases the risk of renal stones. It is important to ensure an adequate intake of dietary calcium. If this is not the case, then calcium supplementation may be required. Occasionally, in patients with very mild hypoparathyroidism, large doses of oral calcium may be enough to correct the serum calcium without vitamin D therapy. Hypocalcaemia secondary to vitamin D deficiency requires vitamin D replacement therapy.

OTHER BONE DISORDERS

Osteoporosis

The aim of treatment in osteoporosis is to reduce fracture risk. There are three components to this:
❏ Reducing falls.
❏ Lifestyle measures.
❏ Drug therapies.

The risk of falling should be minimized through adjustments in the home environment, management of concurrent medical conditions, and occasionally the use of bulky padded hip protectors. Lifestyle changes should include the avoidance of smoking, moderating alcohol consumption, ensuring adequate dietary calcium, and encouraging weight-bearing exercise. Supplemental calcium can be given in tablet form and has been shown to reduce the risk of nonvertebral fractures in the elderly. Before embarking on drug therapies for managing osteoporosis, it is important to correct any hormonal deficiencies or excesses. Corticosteroid drugs should be reduced with the aim of withdrawing them unless medically necessary. Bisphosphonate drugs (alendronate, etidronate, and risedronate) are used commonly to treat osteoporosis. The most common side-effects are gastrointestinal (nausea and diarrhoea). Alendronate is available as a once weekly preparation that needs to be ingested in an

---

Table 61 Acute management of hypocalcaemia

❏ Regular monitoring of serum calcium
❏ Check serum magnesium and replace if low
❏ Cardiac monitoring – high risk of arrhythmias
❏ Intravenous infusion of 20 ml 10% calcium gluconate diluted in 100 ml normal saline over 10 mins
❏ Subsequent infusion of 1100 ml 10% calcium gluconate in 1 litre normal saline over 24 hours

---

upright posture as it can lead to oesophagitis. Other drugs used in managing osteoporosis include:
❏ Hormone replacement therapy (postmenopausal women).
❏ Calcium and vitamin D.
❏ Calcitonin.
❏ Calcitriol.
❏ Fluoride.

Osteoporosis therapy is monitored with 2-yearly measurements of bone mineral density via dual X-ray absorptiometry (DEXA) scanning.

Paget's disease

The bisphosphonates are the treatment of choice in Paget's disease. They are used to control pain, complications, and following fracture. A typical course of treatment is six doses of intravenous pamidronate at weekly intervals. Other bisphosphonates (etidronate, risedronate, tiludronate) can be given orally if symptoms are less acute. Regular 6-monthly measurements of serum alkaline phosphatase provide the best guide to disease activity. Isotope bone scans provide additional information on disease activity.

Ricket's disease and osteomalacia

Where osteomalacia is secondary to underlying disease or toxicity, therapy should be directed at the cause. Management of the vitamin deficiency is through vitamin replacement. Most commonly replacement is given as calciferol (20 µg daily) combined with oral calcium supplementation. Typically symptoms settle quickly, although bone pain and biochemical derangements may persist for several months. Care should be taken to avoid hypercalcaemia. The aim of therapy is to relieve symptoms and return biochemical markers to normal.

CASE 6

A 48-year-old man presents with symptoms of increased thirst, polyuria, and indigestion. On direct questioning he admits to generalized aching in his joints and muscles. He reports no change in weight. His past medical history is unremarkable.

1 What initial investigations should be performed?

Some of his blood test results are shown.

Results (normal range)
Adjusted calcium 3.25 pmol/l (2.10–2.60)
Phosphate 0.79 mmol/l (0.81–1.45)
Parathyroid hormone (PTH) 13 pmol/l (0.9–5.4)

2 What is the likely diagnosis and how should he be managed?

Answers to Case 6 on page 157.

Table 62 Perioperative management of patients with Cushing's syndrome

❑ Metyrapone or ketoconazole given as preparation
❑ Hydrocortisone cover should be given100 mg IV q.d.s. with first dose at induction
❑ Once eating, oral hydrocortisone given (20 mg breakfast, 10 mg lunch, 10 mg teatime)
❑ The dose of hydrocortisone should be halved on recovery (1 week)
❑ Fludrocortisone should be given (100 µg) after bilateral adrenalectomy
❑ Following unilateral adrenalectomy, a Short synacthen test can be performed at 2 weeks to assess steroid requirements
❑ Following unilateral adrenalectomy, the remaining adrenal gland may take up to 2 years to recover

---

MANAGING ADRENAL DISEASE
ADRENAL HORMONE EXCESS
Cushing's syndrome
Iatrogenic Cushing's syndrome

Any unnecessary oral steroid preparations causing Cushing's features should be quickly reduced to physiological doses. For prednisolone, this is a dose of 7.5 mg (reduced by 2.5 mg every 3 days until this dose is achieved). Prednisolone can be converted to hydrocortisone therapy 20 mg daily since this gives less prolonged suppression of the hypo-thalamic–pituitary–adrenal (HPA) axis. The hydrocortisone dose can be reduced by 2.5 mg every 2 weeks. Once the dose is halved, it can be discontinued for 24 hours and a synacthen test can be performed to assess adrenal reserve. If the synacthen test demonstrates a normal response, then the hydrocortisone can be stopped. Patients should be supplied with hydrocortisone in case of emergency for a period of 12 months.

Pituitary-dependent Cushing's disease

The treatment of choice is trans-sphenoidal hypo-physectomy. The cure rate is up to 90% (defined as 9 am cortisol <50 nmol/l, 3 days postoperatively).

The perioperative management of Cushing's syndrome is presented in *Table 62*.

Pituitary radiotherapy can be given as an adjunct to unsuccessful trans-sphenoidal surgery, but the effect on cortisol levels may not be seen for several months or years.

Surgical adrenalectomy is rarely performed for pituitary disease now. The major complication is Nelson's syndrome which typically occurs within the first 1–2 years of adrenalectomy. Features of Nelson's syndrome include:
❑ Hyperpigmentation.
❑ Enlarging pituitary tumour.
❑ Elevated levels of adrenocorticotrophic hormone (ACTH).

Medical treatment to reduce circulating levels is recommended as preoperative preparation since this reduces anaesthetic risk and improves wound healing. Medical treatment is also effective if surgery is contraindicated.

Drug treatment is with either metyrapone, an 11-β-hydroxylase inhibitor (0.25–1 g q.d.s.) or ketoconazole, a P450 enzyme inhibitor (200–400 mg t.d.s.). The dose can be titrated against 24-hour urinary cortisol levels or serum cortisol day curve measurements (blood testing q.d.s.), with the aim of keeping cortisol levels within the normal range. Perioperatively, hydrocortisone replacement should be given.

Adrenal Cushing's disease
The treatment for adrenal Cushing's is surgical removal of the affected adrenal gland. The remaining gland may take several months or even years to recover function so it is important to continue with steroid glucocorticoid and mineralocorticoid replacement until synacthen testing indicates adequate adrenal function. Laparoscopic adrenalectomy has replaced open adrenalectomy in many centres except for large or malignant tumours (see perioperative management, page 139). Where no adrenal tumour is evident, bilateral adrenalectomy or medical therapy should be considered.

Phaeochromocytoma
Optimal management for this condition is medical and then surgical. All patients should receive α- and β-adrenergic blockade prior to surgery. α-blockade should be performed several days before β-blockade. The drug of choice is phenoxybenzamine. It is titrated gradually from 10 mg b.d. to 20 mg q.d.s. The commonest side-effect is nasal stuffiness. Propanolol is then commenced at a dose of 40 mg t.d.s. Intravenous phenoxybenzamine should be given prior to surgery to ensure complete adrenergic blockade.

Surgery may be open or laparoscopic adrenalectomy. Once the tumour is handled, perioperative hypertension may occur. This responds to phentolamine and nitroprusside intravenously. Postoperative hypotension is common and volume replacement with inotropic support is frequently required. Malignant tumours may require long-term α- and β-blockade. Chemotherapy and radiotherapy may give palliative support. The 5-year survival rate is 40%.

Hyperaldosteronism
Surgical treatment
The treatment of choice for aldosterone-secreting adenomas is adrenalectomy. This is increasingly being performed laparoscopically. Patients should receive presurgical treatment with spironolactone (200–400 mg daily). The presurgical response to spironolactone helps to determine those patients who will become normotensive (about 70%). Bilateral nodular hyperplasia does not respond well to surgery.

Medical treatment
Spironolactone is an aldosterone antagonist used in adrenal hyperplasia. This can be combined with other antihypertensive agents, particularly ACE inhibitors and calcium channel blockers. These drugs are also used for patients who are not fit for surgery.

ADRENAL HORMONE DEFICIENCY
The management of adrenal deficiency consists primarily of hormone replacement, monitoring of this replacement, and appropriate education for the patient.

Glucocorticoid (steroid) replacement
In the patient who is acutely unwell, hydrocortisone should be given at a dose of 100 mg 6-hourly intravenously. Chronic management consists of physiological replacement, usually with oral hydrocortisone at a dose of 20 mg daily. Larger patients (>80 kg typically) may require 30 mg daily. A typical regime is 10 mg on waking, 5 mg at noon, and 5 mg in late afternoon (5–6 pm). Prednisolone, cortisone acetate, and dexamethasone are used less frequently since they are longer-acting preparations or have less flexible dosage schedules.

Mineralocorticoid replacement
Most patients with primary adrenocortical insufficiency will require mineralocorticoid replacement (typically 100 μg fludrocortisone given once daily). The presence of postural hypotension and hypokalaemia support the need for mineralocorticoid replacement.

Monitoring hormone replacement
Patients on replacement therapy should receive a regular clinical and biochemical review to include an assessment of the following:
❏ Symptoms.
❏ Weight gain.
❏ Lying and standing blood pressure.
❏ Development of cushingoid features.
❏ Serum electrolytes.
❏ Plasma renin activity (elevated if mineralocorticoid deficiency).
❏ Occasionally, serial daytime cortisol measurements (day curve) to assess for physiological doses of hydrocortisone replacement.

It is important to note that oral hydrocortisone is equivalent to cortisol measured in serum samples. This is not true of other steroid preparations. During severe illness or surgery, patients should be given hydrocortisone intravenously (100 mg q.d.s.) until they are able to return to their maintenance therapy. While recovering, it is common to double their usual oral replacement doses of hydrocortisone for 2–3 days.

Educating patients with adrenocortical deficiency

There are a few important educational issues for the patient on long-term hydrocortisone replacement therapy:

- ❑ A steroid dose should never be missed and if it is, should be given as soon as possible.
- ❑ Some form of identification ahould be carried (e.g. medic-alert bracelet) indicating maintenance steroid replacement.
- ❑ The glucocorticoid dose should be doubled during acute illness, e.g. fever, gastroenteritis, respiratory infection (usually for 2–3 days).
- ❑ If a vomiting illness occurs, medical attention should be sought early.
- ❑ Patients should have a vial of hydrocortisone (100 mg) and a syringe available in case of emergency.

Congenital adrenal hyperplasia (CAH)

Classical CAH

Patients with CAH require hormone replacement with a long-acting steroid, typically prednisolone to switch off ACTH production. Doses of 5–7.5 mg are used, with two-thirds given at bedtime to turn off the nocturnal surge of ACTH. An alternative is dexamethasone (0.5 mg nocte). Fludrocortisone is usually required at a typical daily dose of 100 µg. Patients should be educated to increase steroid dosages during periods of acute illness as for those patients with other forms of adrenocortical insufficiency. The aim of therapy is to restore menstruation where possible and to avoid both adrenal crises and steroid excess.

Nonclassical (late-onset) CAH

Steroid doses may be smaller in this group, e.g. 2.5–5 mg prednisolone given at bedtime. Fludrocortisone is rarely required. Hirsuitism and acne may respond to antiandrogens, e.g. cyproterone (sometimes combined with an oestrogen preparation i.e. Dianette) or, less commonly, spironolactone.

ADRENAL MASSES – INCIDENTALOMAS

There are three indications for surgical removal of an incidentaloma:

- ❑ Size >4 cm.
- ❑ Radiographic appearances suggestive of malignancy.
- ❑ Evidence of excess hormone secretion.

If these criteria are not met, the mass should be followed up with repeat CT scanning at 3, 6, 12, and 24 months to ensure that there is no increase in size or worsening change in appearance.

CASE 7

A 33-year-old woman presents to the Outpatient Clinic with a 6-month history of weight gain, proximal muscle weakness (difficulty in standing from a sitting position), and easy bruising. She has received no drug therapy. On examination she has a round plethoric face, central obesity, a prominent 'buffalo hump', with purple striae over her anterior abdominal wall. Her blood pressure is elevated (155/95 mmHg). Cushing's syndrome is suspected, and a screening test is organized followed by other diagnostic investigations. The results are shown.

Results (normal range)
24-hour urinary cortisol 877 nmol/24 hr (<280 nmol/24 hr)
Low-dose dexamethasone suppression test (0.5 mg dexamethasone given 6 hourly for 48 hours): plasma cortisol 723 nmol/l (<100 nmol/l)
Plasma adrenocorticotrophic hormone (ACTH) 0.1 pmol/l (3.3–15.4)
Pituitary magnetic resonance imaging (MRI) scan: normal

1 What is the diagnosis?
2 What is the treatment?

Answers to Case 7 on page 157.

CASE 8

A 28-year-old man presents to his General Practitioner with anorexia, weakness, and vomiting. His symptoms have been present intermittently for several months. He says that he has lost 20 kg in weight over this period. He has felt overwhelmingly fatigued and has to stop participating in weekly football matches because of this. His only medication is levothyroxine 100 µg once daily for previous hypothyroidism.

On examination he is very thin (body mass index [BMI] 29) but tanned. He has profound generalized muscle weakness. He has excessive pigmentation overlying his knees and elbows.

1 What is the diagnosis and what investigation does he require?
2 What treatment should be recommended?

Answers to Case 8 on page 158.

MANAGING PITUITARY DISEASE
PITUITARY HORMONE EXCESS
Prolactinoma

Prolactinomas are amenable to pharmacological treatment because of the availability of dopamine agonists that decrease the secretion and size of the tumour. Treatment is required for neurological symptoms, hypogonadism, or other symptoms due to hyperprolactinaemia. A tumour extending outside of the sella and abutting or elevating the optic chiasm, or invading the cavernous or sphenoid is likely to continue to grow and eventually cause neurological symptoms. Patients with symptoms of hypogonadism or troublesome galactorrhoea and patients with macroprolactinomas should receive dopamine agonist therapy.

Dopamine agonists decrease prolactin (PRL) secretion and reduce the size of the lactotroph adenoma in > 90% of patients. The fall in serum PRL typically occurs within the first 2–3 weeks of therapy.

The decrease in adenoma size is detected by imaging between 6 weeks and 6 months after initiation of treatment; in some patients, however, a decrease is not apparent for 6 months. These benefits also occur in patients who have impaired visual fields before therapy. Visual and pituitary dysfunction often return to normal. There is recovery of menses and fertility in women, and of testosterone secretion, sperm count, and erectile function in men. Patients with macroadenomas who are hypothyroid and/or hypoadrenal may also have a return of these functions to normal.

The principal side-effects of dopamine agonist drugs are nausea, postural hypotension, and mental fogginess. Side-effects are more likely to occur when treatment is initiated or the dose is increased. They can be avoided in most patients by starting with a small dose and by giving it with food or at bedtime. The dose should then be increased gradually. Several dopamine agonists are effective:

❑ Cabergoline is the best initial choice in most circumstances, because it is most likely to be effective and least likely to cause side-effects. The initial dose should be 0.25 mg twice a week or 0.5 mg once weekly.
❑ For a woman who wishes to become pregnant, bromocriptine is a better first-line agent because there is more evidence that it does not cause birth defects. Bromocriptine should be started at a dose of 1.25 mg after dinner or at bedtime for 1 week, then increased to 1.25 mg twice a day (after breakfast and after dinner or at bedtime).
❑ Quinagolide is an alternative choice, used more widely on the European mainland.

Monitoring dopamine agonist therapy

After 1 month of therapy, the patient should be evaluated for side-effects and serum PRL should be measured. Subsequent treatment depends upon the response. With macroprolactinomas, the dose should be increased monthly. If vision was abnormal before therapy, it should be reassessed within 1 month, although improvement may occur within a few days. Magnetic resonance imaging (MRI) should be repeated in 6–12 months to determine if the size of the adenoma has decreased.

The drug should be stopped if the patient becomes pregnant. If no adenoma is visualized, it may be possible to try a discontinuation of therapy a few years after initiation, but the serum PRL should be monitored. After the menopause, if there is a microprolactinoma present, the drug can be discontinued and the serum

PRL concentration can be allowed to rise up to 3000 mU/l. If the patient cannot tolerate the first agonist tried or the adenoma does not respond to it, an alternative agonist should be suggested.

Other treatments

If dopamine agonist therapy is not effective in a patient with a microadenoma, oestrogen and progesterone replacement should be considered in a woman who does not wish to conceive. This may be a reasonable option for women with hyperprolactinaemia and amenorrhoea due to antipsychotic agents. It can be given in the form of an oral contraceptive preparation. PRL should be measured periodically as there is a risk of increased tumour size on oestrogen.

Trans-sphenoidal surgery

Surgical treatment should be considered when:
- ❏ Dopamine agonist treatment has been unsuccessful in lowering the serum PRL concentration or size of the adenoma, and symptoms or signs due to hyperprolactinaemia or adenoma size persist during treatment.
- ❏ A woman has a giant prolactinoma e.g. >3 cm, and wishes to become pregnant, since the adenoma may increase to a clinically important size during pregnancy.

The adenoma and hyperprolactinaemia may recur within several years after surgery. This is more likely with larger tumours. It is important to follow up serum PRL levels for several years postsurgery.

Radiotherapy

Radiotherapy directed at the pituitary fossa can be considered where there is residual tumour following surgery. Side-effects include nausea, lassitude, loss of taste and smell, and loss of scalp hair at the radiation portals during and shortly after the treatment. There is also a 50% chance of loss of anterior pituitary hormone secretion during the subsequent 10 years after pituitary radiotherapy.

Treatment of hyperprolactinaemia unrelated to prolactinoma

Treatment depends on the cause of the hyperprolactinaemia:
- ❏ Secondary to hypothalamic and pituitary disease. If removal of the adenoma or mass is not possible, the hyperprolactinaemia should be treated with a dopamine agonist.
- ❏ Drug-induced. If the drug cannot be discontinued because it is essential, and no substitute can be found, the resulting hypogonadism can be treated with the appropriate sex steroid. Dopamine agonist therapy might counteract the dopamine antagonist property of the antipsychotic drug.
- ❏ Secondary to hypothyroidism. If hyperprolactinaemia is solely the result of hypothyroidism, it will settle on thyroxine replacement.
- ❏ Treatment of galactorrhoea with normal PRL. For the unusual patient whose galactorrhoea occurs spontaneously and to a degree that causes staining of the clothes, treatment with a low dose of a dopamine agonist, such as 0.25 mg of cabergoline twice a week, will reduce the PRL concentration to below normal and should reduce or eliminate the galactorrhoea.

ACTH-secreting adenoma
(See management of Cushing's disease, page 139)

TSH-secreting adenoma

Pituitary surgery is the treatment of choice for a TSH-secreting pituitary adenoma. Adjunctive radiotherapy is often required. Somatostatin analogues, e.g. octreotide, can reduce TSH levels and may shrink the tumour. They are a useful preoperative treatment. Treatment with antithyroid drugs should be avoided as this leads to increased TSH secretion in many patients. Beta-blockers such as propanolol may give symptomatic relief. Thyroid surgery should be reserved for patients with symptomatic thyroid goitres in whom other therapy has failed.

Acromegaly (growth hormone [GH]-secreting adenoma)

Surgical resection

Surgery is the treatment of choice for patients with acromegaly. It should be offered for patients with small pituitary adenomas and for large but still resectable tumours, particularly where it is causing visual impairment. Surgery can also be considered for large adenomas that are not entirely accessible surgically, with the goal of removing a sufficient mass of tissue to enlarge the options for subsequent adjuvant therapy. When performed by the most experienced pituitary neurosurgeons, GH secretion falls to normal in about 80% of patients with microadenomas. The success rate is lower in patients with macroadenomas (<50%). After trans-sphenoidal surgery, serum GH concentration typically falls to normal within 1–2 hours, depending upon the degree of elevation. Serum insulin-like growth factor-1 (IGF-1) concentration often falls to normal in 7–10 days, but can remain high for several months before declining to normal. Vision and headaches can improve in days. Approximately 3–10 of patients in whom the operation is initially successful, as determined by normal basal and normal postglucose serum GH concentrations, have a recurrence several years or more after surgery. The mortality rate is very low (<1%) even in patients with large adenomas.

Drug treatment

Pharmacological treatment is usually used in acromagaly as a secondary treatment when surgery has not reduced GH and IGF-1 levels to normal. Its role in primary treatment has not yet been clearly established. It can be used for patients who have unacceptable surgical risk, refuse surgery, or have adenomas that are surgically inaccessible.

Somatostatin analogues

Somatostatin analogues (e.g. octreotide and lanreotide) inhibit GH secretion more effectively than endogenous somatostatin and are often effective in reducing elevated serum GH concentrations in acromegaly. Octreotide is available in short- and long-acting forms in both Europe and the US; lanreotide is available in two long-acting forms in Europe. The initial dose of the short-acting form of octreotide is 100 µg subcutaneously every 8 hours. If the serum IGF-1 concentration does not decrease to normal within 1–2 months, the dose can be increased gradually, to a maximum of 500 µg every 8 hours.

The long-acting form of octreotide is given as a deep intramuscular injection once a month. The initial dose is 20 mg once a month. If the serum IGF-1 concentration does not decrease to normal within 2 months, the dose can be increased to 30 mg and then to 40 mg a month. Lanreotide is available in an intramuscular form, which is given as 30 mg every 7–14 days, and a deep subcutaneous form which is given as 60–120 mg every 4 weeks.

Efficacy should be judged by normalization of the serum GH and IGF-1 concentrations, which should eventually be followed by regression of the soft tissue manifestations of acromegaly and by adenoma size. Medical treatment normalizes IGF-1 in one-third to two-thirds of patients. Serum IGF-1 is associated with an improvement in the clinical manifestations of

acromegaly, including soft tissue swelling, carpal tunnel syndrome, and snoring. Left ventricular mass decreases and left ventricular function improves concomitantly with the fall of serum GH and IGF-1 levels. About 30% of patients have a significant decrease in tumour size. A disadvantage of somatostatin analogues is their high cost. They are generally well tolerated but there are some important side-effects:

❑ Nausea.
❑ Abdominal discomfort.
❑ Bloating.
❑ Loose stools.
❑ Mild glucose intolerance rarely occurs.
❑ Cholesterol gallstones (25%).

Dopamine agonists

Dopamine agonists such as cabergoline or bromocriptine may inhibit GH secretion in patients with acromegaly and have the advantage over other treatments that they are taken orally. The initial dose of cabergoline should be 0.5 mg once a week or 0.25 mg twice a week. The dose should be increased, if necessary, to 1.0 mg twice a week.

Cabergoline is less effective than somatostatin analogues in reducing IGF-1 but may be effective in up to one-third of patients. Bromocriptine appears to be less effective than cabergoline.

GH receptor antagonist

Pegvisomant is a GH receptor antagonist administered as a daily subcutaneous injection. The initial daily dose is 10 mg. The serum IGF-1 concentration should be measured every 4–6 weeks and the dose adjusted, in 5 mg increments, to a maximum of 30 mg/day, to keep the serum IGF-1 within the normal range. Because the drug does not inhibit GH secretion, GH cannot be used to monitor the effectiveness of treatment. A very large number of patients (>95%) achieve normal IGF-1 levels with this treatment. Patients who are treated should be monitored by liver function tests once a month during the first 6 months of treatment. Tumour size may, however, increase and patients should have adenoma size assessed by MRI annually.

Radiotherapy

Radiotherapy may be used in patients whose disease is not controlled by surgery or medical therapy. The frequency of neurological side-effects may be great, and it is contraindicated in patients with suprasellar tumour extension, because the optic tracts may lie in the radiation field.

Adenoma growth is invariably arrested, but the decline in GH secretion is very slow (sometimes >10 years). Normalization of the serum IGF-1 concentration is about 50% in 10 years. Within 10 years, about 50% of patients treated with pituitary radiation develop deficiency of one or more pituitary hormones. Second intracranial tumours have been reported in up to 1.7% of patients within the first 10 years after pituitary radiation.

Stereotactic radiotherapy is a technique performed in a limited number of specialized centres but may give improved results over standard radiotherapy. Follow-up investigations for the patient with acromegaly are presented in *Table 63*.

Gonadotrophin and nonfunctioning pituitary adenomas

These tumours are frequently not detected until they become sufficiently large to cause neurological symptoms, most often impaired vision due to pressure on the optic chiasm. Treatment to relieve those symptoms must be instituted promptly. Standard treatment is usually trans-sphenoidal surgery, occasionally followed by radiation. Trans-sphenoidal surgery reduces the size of the adenoma and its hormonal hypersecretion in more than 90% of cases. It also improves vision in about 70%.

Serious complications of trans-sphenoidal surgery in the immediate postoperative period occur in <5% of patients. These are worsening vision, haemorrhage, and meningitis. A common postoperative problem is instability of antidiuretic hormone (ADH) secretion, which can include diabetes insipidus or the syndrome of inappropriate antidiuretic hormone secretion (SIADH) lasting several days. Occasionally, permanent diabetes insipidus can occur. The risk of complications is inversely proportional to the experience of the surgeon in performing trans-sphenoidal surgery.

Monitoring of pituitary tumours

For short-term monitoring, the patient should be evaluated for the amount of residual adenoma (usually by MRI), visual acuity and visual fields, and pituitary hormone function within 2 months of surgery. This evaluation should include measurements of serum thyroxine, early morning serum cortisol 48 hours after discontinuation, serum testosterone (men) or oestradiol (premenopausal women), and 24-hour urine volume if the patient has significant nocturia. Long-term monitoring should include testing every 6–12 months initially, to detect growth of residual adenoma tissue and the adequacy of hormonal replacement. Vision should also be periodically evaluated if it was affected by the adenoma.

Radiotherapy is useful in preventing regrowth of a pituitary adenoma when an MRI performed 6–12 months after surgery shows substantial residual adenoma tissue that poses a significant neurological risk. It is also useful when residual adenoma tissue shows progressive growth in the months or years after surgery. It can be used as primary therapy in selected patients whose adenomas are sufficiently large to threaten the optic chiasm but are not causing visual impairment or other neurological symptoms.

Table 63 Follow-up investigations for patients with acromegaly

❏ IGF-1 levels and an assessment of GH response to a glucose tolerance test should be carried out at regular intervals according to response
❏ MRI should be repeated annually for the first few years after any initial treatment
❏ Visual field assessment is indicated for patients whose adenomas threaten the optic chiasm
❏ Colonoscopy should be carried out at 3–4 year intervals in patients over 50 years old
❏ Cardiovascular evaluation should be performed regularly and hypertension and cardiac failure treated aggressively

Gonadotrophin or nonfunctioning adenomas that are asymptomatic and not an immediate threat to vision may not require treatment. An increasing number of nonfunctioning adenomas are detected as incidental findings when MRI is performed for other reasons. However, hormonal deficiencies should still be replaced, and re-evaluation of adenoma size and function of the nonadenomatous pituitary should be performed at yearly intervals.

Other sellar masses

Management of lesions other than pituitary adenomas in the region of the sellar typically consists of surgical removal with attention paid to monitoring of pituitary function and tumour growth. Detailed discussion of the management of nonendocrine sellar masses is not covered in this text.

PITUITARY HORMONE DEFICIENCY

ACTH

Lack of ACTH primarily induces cortisol deficiency. Treatment consists of the administration of a glucocorticoid such as hydrocortisone to mimic the normal pattern of cortisol secretion. Unlike the situation in primary adrenal insufficiency, mineralocorticoid replacement is rarely necessary in hypopituitarism. An unusual side-effect of glucocorticoid replacement is the unmasking of underlying central diabetes insipidus; correction of cortisol deficiency can increase the blood pressure and renal blood flow, and, in patients with partial diabetes insipidus, reduce the secretion of ADH.

TSH

TSH deficiency results in thyroxine deficiency, and is treated with thyroxine replacement. The goal of therapy should be a normal serum T4 value. Thyroxine should not be administered until adrenal function, including ACTH reserve, has been evaluated and either found to be normal or treated. Thyroxine increases the clearance of cortisol and increases the severity of cortisol deficiency.

Unlike primary hypothyroidism, measurement of serum TSH cannot be used as a guide to the adequacy of L-thyroxine replacement therapy. The treatment goal should be a serum T4 concentration in the middle or upper end of the normal range.

Luteinizing hormone [LH]/ follicle stimulating hormone [FSH]

In men

Testosterone replacement is required for men who have hypogonadism and who are not interested in fertility. The choice of treatment does not differ from that in men with primary hypogonadism. Serum LH measurements cannot be used to monitor the adequacy of therapy. This can be achieved by measurements of serum testosterone.

Men with secondary hypogonadism who wish to become fertile can be treated with gonadotrophins (LH and FSH) if they have pituitary disease, or with either gonadotrophins or gonadotrophin releasing hormone (GnRH) if they have hypothalamic disease.

In women

Premenopausal women who are not interested in fertility can be treated with oestrogen and progesterone replacement therapy (typically a low-dose contraceptive pill). Women who wish to become fertile may be treated with pulsatile GnRH or gonadotrophins.

Serum androgen concentrations in women with hypopituitarism are significantly lower than those in normal control women There is some evidence that low dose testosterone increases bone mineral density, some aspects of mood, sexual function, and quality of life, as assessed by questionnaires. This therapy may be considered in selected individuals.

GH

Deficiency of GH in childhood leads to short stature and GH replacement is essential.

Patients who develop GH deficiency in adulthood have unfavourable serum lipid profiles, increased body fat, decreased muscle mass, decreased bone mineral density, and a diminished sense of well being. There is substantial evidence that GH treatment in these patients increases muscle mass, reduces body fat, and improves quality of life.

Recombinant human growth hormone is licensed for use in adults who are deficient in GH. In the UK its use is recommended for those whose symptoms lead to a significantly impaired quality of life as measured by a validated questionnaire.

GH is administered by subcutaneous injection once a day, usually in the evening. The goal is to keep the serum IGF-1 concentration within the middle of the age-adjusted normal range. A typical daily dose is 10 µg/kg body weight. A starting dose of 2–5 µg/kg body weight is recommended. The daily dose should be increased in stepwise increments at 2-month intervals until it is normal. If side-effects occur or the serum IGF-1 concentration increases to above normal at any dose, the dose should be decreased.

The most common side-effects of GH treatment in adults with hypopituitarism are:

❑ Peripheral oedema.
❑ Arthralgia.
❑ Carpal tunnel syndrome.
❑ Paraesthesiae.
❑ Worsening of glucose tolerance.

Active malignancy is considered to be a contraindication to GH treatment, because of the theoretical possibility that the treatment could stimulate tumour growth. No direct evidence is yet available. UK recommendations are that quality of life assessment should be repeated at 6 months and, if there is no improvement, then GH replacement should be discontinued.

PRL

The only known presentation of prolactin deficiency is the inability to lactate after delivery (for which there is currently no available treatment).

ADH (diabetes insipidus [DI])

Cranial DI

Since the primary problem in cranial DI is deficient secretion of ADH, control of the polyuria can be achieved by hormone replacement with desmopressin. The initial aim of therapy is to reduce nocturia, thereby providing adequate sleep; after this is achieved, one aims for control of the diuresis during the day. In patients with partial DI who are passing <4 litres of urine per day, adequate fluid replacement may be all that is required.

Desmopressin is in liquid form that is usually administered intranasally and in an oral tablet form. The intranasal preparation can be blown into the nose by the patient with a curved, dose-calibrated small plastic tube or delivered with a nasal spray. An initial dose of 5 µg at bedtime can be titrated upward in 5 µg increments, depending upon the response of the nocturia, and then additional daytime doses added. The daily maintenance dose is about 5–20 µg once or twice a day. The desmopressin metered spray bottle is currently used more commonly than the rhinal catheter because of greater convenience of administration. The usual daily maintenance dose is 10–20 µg intranasally once or twice a day. An oral

tablet preparation of desmopressin is also available. The 0.1 mg tablet is the equivalent of 2.5–5 µg of the nasal spray. However, because the oral dose cannot be precisely predicted from a previous nasal dose, transferring of patients requires re-titration. The initial dose of the tablet form is 0.05 mg. The usual daily maintenance dose ranges from 0.1 mg to 0.8 mg in divided doses but may be as high as 1.2 mg/day.

The main concern with desmopressin replacement is water retention and the development of hyponatraemia. Patients with this disorder are generally not in danger of marked fluid loss and hypernatraemia as long as their thirst mechanism is intact. However, once desmopressin is given, the patient has nonsuppressible ADH activity and may be unable to excrete ingested water normally. This problem can be avoided by giving the minimum dose that is required to control the polyuria. The first dose (5–10 µg of the nasal spray or 0.1 or 0.2 mg tablet) is usually given in the late evening to control the most troubling symptom of nocturia. The size of, and necessity for, a daytime dose can then be determined by the effectiveness of the evening dose. If, for example, polyuria does not recur until noon, then one-half the evening dose may be sufficient at that time.

Other treatment for DI

Chlorpropramide increases the renal response to ADH. The usual dose is 125–250 mg, once or twice a day and is effective in partial DI but is rarely used. Thiazide diuretics and nonsteroidal anti-inflammatory drugs (NSAIDs) (indomethacin) can be used with other agents in central DI. The efficacy of a NSAIDs is dependent upon the inhibition of renal prostaglandin synthesis. This has the effect of increasing concentrating ability, since prostaglandins normally antagonize the action of ADH.

Nephrogenic DI

Correcting the underlying disorder (e.g. hypercalcaemia) or discontinuing the offending drug (e.g. lithium) should be the first line of therapy. In hereditary cases, a low dose of thiazide diuretic should be used. If this is unhelpful, then indomethacin can be added. In some cases it may be necessary to try high doses of desmopressin.

> *All patients with DI requiring therapy should be reviewed on a regular basis with attention paid to symptoms, serum sodium, and osmolarity.*

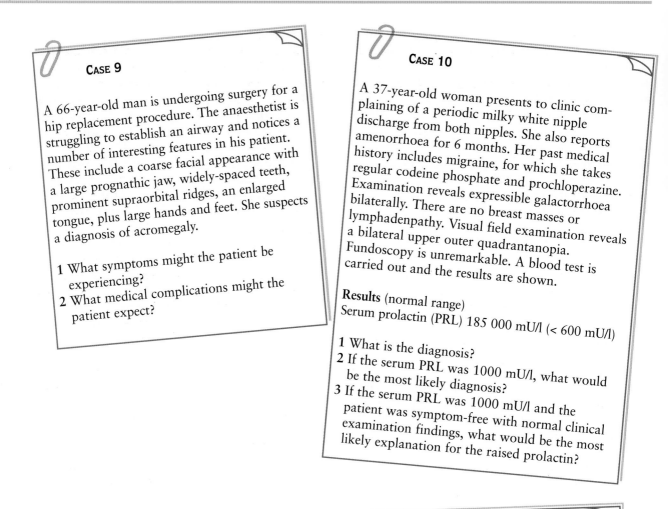

CASE 9

A 66-year-old man is undergoing surgery for a hip replacement procedure. The anaesthetist is struggling to establish an airway and notices a number of interesting features in his patient. These include a coarse facial appearance with a large prognathic jaw, widely-spaced teeth, prominent supraorbital ridges, an enlarged tongue, plus large hands and feet. She suspects a diagnosis of acromegaly.

1 What symptoms might the patient be experiencing?
2 What medical complications might the patient expect?

CASE 10

A 37-year-old woman presents to clinic complaining of a periodic milky white nipple discharge from both nipples. She also reports amenorrhoea for 6 months. Her past medical history includes migraine, for which she takes regular codeine phosphate and prochloperazine. Examination reveals expressible galactorrhoea bilaterally. There are no breast masses or lymphadenpathy. Visual field examination reveals a bilateral upper outer quadrantanopia. Fundoscopy is unremarkable. A blood test is carried out and the results are shown.

Results (normal range)
Serum prolactin (PRL) 185 000 mU/l (< 600 mU/l)

1 What is the diagnosis?
2 If the serum PRL was 1000 mU/l, what would be the most likely diagnosis?
3 If the serum PRL was 1000 mU/l and the patient was symptom-free with normal clinical examination findings, what would be the most likely explanation for the raised prolactin?

CASE 11

A 76-year-old man presents to the Accident & Emergency Department feeling unwell. He has been sent to hospital by his daughter who complains that he is 'off his legs'. He complains of weakness, fatigue, and feeling cold. He complains of weight loss but is not sure how much. On examination he is pale with cool peripheries. His blood pressure is low (90/55 mmHg), his pulse is 58 bpm. There is a paucity of body hair and there is generalized muscle weakness. A number of blood tests are carried out. His hormone profile is shown.

Results (normal range)
Free T4 3.2 pmol/l (10.3–24.5)
Thyroid stimulating hormone (TSH) 1.2 nmol/l (0.4–4.0)
Testosterone 1.1 nmol/l (9–42)

1 What is the most likely diagnosis?
2 What investigation should be carried out urgently?
3 How should this man's missing hormones be replaced?

Answers to Cases 9, 10, & 11 on page 158.

MANAGING METABOLIC DISEASE
GASTROINTESTINAL NEUROENDOCRINE TUMOURS

Insulinoma

Localized insulinomas should be surgically removed. For patients whose insulinoma cannot be located during pancreatic exploration or who are not candidates for surgery, diazoxide therapy is used to medically manage the patients. For patients with metastatic insulinoma, resection of isolated hepatic metastases along with the primary tumour can be performed although this is rarely curative. Other treatment options include somatostatin analogues, interferon-alpha, chemoembolization, and systemic chemotherapy.

Glucagonoma

For the minority of cases in which the tumour remains localized at the time of diagnosis, resection of the primary pancreatic tumour is indicated. Resection results in a complete cure rate of only about 30%. Because patients with glucagonoma syndrome suffer from a prolonged catabolic state, nutritional support may be an important component of therapy. Other approaches to the treatment of hepatic metastases include the use of radiofrequency ablation (RFA) and cryoablation, either alone or in conjunction with surgical debulking. Orthotopic liver transplantation has been performed in a small number of patients with islet cell tumours. Embolization and chemo-embolization of liver metastases may increase life expectancy and reduce symptoms.

The somatostatin analogue octreotide inhibits hormone secretion and is the first-line therapy for symptomatic glucagonoma syndrome in patients with unresectable tumours. Therapy is initiated with 50 µg subcutaneously three times a day, and the dose is increased gradually as needed to control symptoms Long-acting forms of octreotide are now more frequently used. Interferon-alpha has also been effective in controlling symptoms in patients who are resistant to octreotide therapy. Systemic chemotherapy is also used. Many patients are able to experience prolonged survival with a combination of medical and surgical therapies for periods in excess of 5 years.

Zollinger-Ellison syndrome (ZES)

Medical therapy is the current standard of care for most patients with ZES as part of the MEN Type 1 syndrome. The goal of medical management is to limit the clinical manifestations and complications. For any patient with a sporadic gastrinoma and without evidence of metastatic spread of disease, exploratory laparotomy should be performed since it offers the possibility of cure and decreases the need for medical therapy. Cure rates of one-third have been reported. Treatments for metastatic disease are of limited benefit and, whenever possible, the patient should participate in the decision. Available therapeutic options include somatostatin analogues, interferon-alpha, cytotoxic chemotherapy, surgical resection of hepatic metastases, and hepatic arterial chemoembolization.

Carcinoid syndrome

The treatment of choice for a patient who has a localized carcinoid tumour is surgery. For patients with metastatic disease and the carcinoid syndrome, symptomatic therapies are used. The patient should be advised to avoid factors that induce flushing episodes, such as alcohol ingestion or specific forms of physical activity. Mild diarrhoea may respond to codeine phosphate. Asthma can be treated with theophylline or β-agonists. The most effective medical therapy is the somatostatin analogue octreotide, given daily subcutaneously or, now more frequently, intramuscularly as a longer-acting preparation monthly.

Curative surgery can be offered only to the rare patient with resectable nodal, hepatic, or with an isolated brain metastasis. Surgical procedures in patients with carcinoid syndrome are potentially hazardous. Resection of hepatic metastases can palliate symptoms of hormonal hypersecretion and may result in long-term survival. Other treatments for hepatic metastases are RFA, cryoablation, liver transplantation, interferon-alpha, chemotherapy, embolization, and chemoembolization.

Carcinoid crisis

Profound flushing, extreme changes in blood pressure, bronchoconstriction, arrhythmias, confusion, and drowsiness may occur spontaneously after palpation of tumour during induction of anaesthesia. The crisis may be fatal. The blood pressure should be supported by infusion of plasma and octreotide should be administered. Octreotide should also be given prior to general anaesthesia and hepatic artery embolization, to prevent carcinoid crisis.

Carcinoid tumours are characterized by slow growth. The 5-year survival for localized tumours is 95%. With widely metastatic tumours, the mean survival rates are <2 years.

Vasointestinal peptide (VIP)oma

Treatment of a patient with a VIPoma requires adequate replacement of fluid losses and correction of electrolyte abnormalities before surgical removal of localized tumour. Octreotide is the treatment of choice to control diarrhoea. For metastatic disease, octreotide is the first-line therapy for symptomatic disease in patients with unresectable tumours. Surgical resection of hepatic metastases can palliate symptoms and may improve survival. RFA, cryoablation, liver transplantation, embolization, and chemoembolization have been used for liver metastases. Interferon-alpha has been used as an adjunctive therapy. Chemotherapy is rarely useful. A favourable prognosis is associated with small tumours (<4 cm), the absence of metastasis, and young age.

Somatostatinoma

As with other neuroendocrine tumours, surgical resection is the treatment of choice. 75% of patients have metastatic disease at presentation. Resection of isolated hepatic metastases and liver transplantation for widespread hepatic metastases may be effective. Debulking surgery can provide symptomatic relief and extended survival. RFA and cryoablation, embolization, and chemoembolization for liver metastases are also used. Octreotide is the first-line therapy for symptomatic disease in patients with unresectable tumours. Interferon-alfa and systemic chemotherapy are occasionally added. The 5-year survival rates in metastaic disease have been reported as 15–50%.

ELECTROLYTE ABNORMALITIES
Hyponatraemia

The management of hyponatraemia depends upon the underlying cause. In addition to management of the underlying problem, the following therapeutic approaches are recommended.

Renal or nonrenal salt loss
This can be treated with dietary salt replacement, which can be given in tablet form if required. Intravenous saline may be required in patients who are clinically dehydrated.

Dilutional hyponatraemia in organ failure and SIADH
Fluid should be restricted to 0.5–1.0 l/day. Occasionally hypertonic (3%) saline should be used intravenously in patients with profound hyponatraemia. Rapid correction of hyponatraemia (>0.5 mmol/h) should be avoided as there is a risk of potentially fatal central pontine myelinolysis. In chronic SIADH where fluid restriction is problematic or ineffective, oral demeclocycline can be used. This induces a nephrogenic DI.

RENAL TUBULAR ABNORMALITIES
Bartter's syndrome
Oral potassium replacement coupled with an NSAID (indomethacin 2–5 mg/day) is usually effective in correcting potassium and alleviating symptoms. Potassium sparing diuretics are sometimes used.

Gitelman's syndrome
Oral potassium and magnesium replacement is the mainstay of treatment. Potassium sparing diuretics are sometimes used.

Liddles's syndrome
Amiloride is the treatment of choice for the hypokalaemia and hypertension.

INHERITED ENDOCRINE SYNDROMES
Multiple endocrine neoplasia (MEN) Type 1
Routine screening should be carried out in the following patients:
- Anyone with two MEN-1 tumours.
- First-degree relatives of MEN-1 patients.
- Young patients with primary hyperparathyroidism (<50 years).
- Anyone with a pancreatic endocrine tumour.

Screening tests should include the following:
- Serum calcium.
- PRL.
- Fasting gastrin.

Management of patients with this condition is as for each complication. Most die from pancreatic malignancy.

MEN Type 2
Routine genetic screening should be carried out in first-degree relatives with a known mutation and in first- and second-degree relatives of patients with no mutation. Most genetic mutations are detectable.

In those with a genetic mutation, annual biochemical testing should be carried out:

❑ Calcitonin +/- pentagastrin test.
❑ Serum calcium.
❑ Urine catecholamines.

In addition, MRI imaging of the adrenal glands should be carried out every 3 years.

Medullary thyroid cancer is managed with total thyroidectomy and removal of locally involved lymph glands. This is followed by postoperative thyroxine replacement. Regular measurement of calcitonin is useful in detecting recurrence or metastases. MRI imaging and octreotide scanning are also used to detect recurrence.

Other complications are managed as described elsewhere. Removal of an adrenal phaeochromocytoma should precede thyroidectomy.

DYSLIPIDAEMIA

Hypercholesterolaemia is an important risk factor for the development of coronary heart disease and other circulatory disease; reducing elevated cholesterol reduces this risk for those with and without established coronary heart disease. Target cholesterol levels have been established for many groups of patients, particularly those with established circulatory disease and those at high risk of cardiovascular disease. Risk charts indicating the risk of developing cardiovascular disease and guidelines for treatment targets have been produced and updated by Joint British Societies and are published in the British National Formulary. This section aims to summarize the treatments available for the management of dyslipidaemias, and assumes that secondary causes have been addressed. *Table 64* presents the management targets for patients with elevated low-density lipoprotein (LDL)-cholesterol alone or with elevated triglycerides, and for those with elevated triglycerides alone.

In severe hypercholesterolaemia or hypertriglyceridaemia, recurrent plasmaphoresis may be required. This is more commonly required in severe inherited dyslipidaemias where drugs are less effective.

Statins (HMG CoA reductase inhibitors)
This group of drugs inhibits cholesterol synthesis in the liver and has proved highly effective in clinical trials in reducing LDL- and total cholesterol levels, with subsequent reductions in death and atherosclerotic

---

Table 64 Management targets for patients with elevated low-density lipoprotein (LDL)-cholesterol alone or with elevated triglycerides, and for those with elevated triglycerides alone

LDL-cholesterol +/– elevated triglycerides

❑ Diet: all patients should receive dietary advice. Fat ingestion should be low (<30% daily energy inake). Saturated fat intake should be low (<30% total fat consumption). Fresh fruit and vegetables should be eaten daily (>4 portions). The intake of dietary fibre should be encouraged. Alcohol consumption should not be excessive (<21 units/week)
❑ Weight reduction in overweight patients
❑ Increased physical activity (30 minutes of exercise inducing breathlessness daily)
❑ Smoking cessation
❑ Management of other cardiovascular risk factors (blood pressure, diabetes control)
❑ Statin therapy
❑ Ezetimibe
❑ Bile acid sequestrants
❑ Nicotinic acid derivatives
❑ Fibrates

Elevated triglycerides alone

❑ Diet
❑ Weight reduction in overweight patients
❑ Increased physical activity
❑ Smoking cessation
❑ Management of other cardiovascular risk factors
❑ Fibrates
❑ Nicotinic acid derivatives
❑ Maxepa

---

disease events. It includes atorvastatin, fluvastatin, pravastatin, rosuvastatin, and simvastatin. The effect on triglyceride levels is less. Atorvastatin and rosuvastatin appear more potent in reducing LDL-cholesterol and triglyceride levels.

Statins can cause a hepatitis and myositis-like state in some individuals. Liver function tests and creatinine kinase levels should be measured before therapy, at 3 months following therapy, and annually thereafter. They should also be measured in symptomatic patients. Muscles can become swollen or tender and rhabdomyolysis can occur. This is more common in patients on fibrates or cyclosporin and when combined with renal impairment or untreated hypothyroidism. The drug should be stopped if liver alanine aminotransferase (ALT) levels rise significantly (>2–3× above normal) or if muscle symptoms are accompanied by a rise in creatinine kinase (CK) (usually >10×). Statins interact with a wide range of other drugs; each differs, so care must be taken when coprescribing.

Fibrates

This group of drugs acts mainly by decreasing triglycerides and raising high-density lipoprotein (HDL)-cholesterol through increased lipoprotein lipase activity. They have variable effects on reducing LDL-cholesterol. The drugs are bezafibrate, ciprofibrate, fenofibrate, and gemfibrozil. They are most effective in treating hypertriglyceridaemia or mixed hyperlipidaemias. They can cause myositis and rhabdomyolysis. This risk dramatically increases when combined with a statin.

Bile acid sequestrants

Cholestyramine and colestipol are anion-exchange resins that bind bile acids, preventing their reabsorption. This results in increased conversion of cholesterol to bile acids and reduced LDL-cholesterol. There may, however, be an increase in serum triglycerides. They are frequently used as an adjunt to statins. Side-effects include nausea, abdominal discomfort, and constipation and doses should be titrated upwards gradually. They are licensed for use in pregnancy.

Nicotinic acid and its derivatives

These drugs inhibit synthesis of both triglycerides and cholesterol. They form the most effective medication for increasing HDL-cholesterol and reducing triglycerides. Side-effects are common with nicotinic acid (flushing and dyspepsia). Acipimox is a less potent derivative with fewer side-effects.

Ezetimibe

This is an intestinal inhibitor of cholesterol that can be combined with a statin drug for increased reduction in serum cholesterol. It is being used increasingly since, unlike fibrates, it does not appear to potentiate the myositis associated with statin use.

MANAGING REPRODUCTIVE DISEASE
REPRODUCTIVE HORMONE EXCESS
Polycystic ovarian syndrome (PCOS)

Management of PCOS depends upon the presenting symptoms. However, weight loss in obese patients will reduce both insulin resistance and hyperandrogenism so usually has a positive impact on hirsuitism, menstrual regularity, and subfertility. Other therapies are specific to the presenting problem and are detailed below.

Oral therapies for hirsuitism are often only partially effective but there are a number of treatments worth trying:

❑ Oral contraceptive pill (OCP). This increases sex hormone-binding globulin (SHBG) levels and reduces free androgen concentration.
❑ Antiandrogens:
  ❑ Dianette. This is a combination of an OCP with low-dose cyproterone acetate (2 mg), an antiandrogen.
  ❑ Cyproterone (up to 100 mg) added cyclically (days 5–14) to an OCP.
  ❑ Spironolactone (usually 50 mg twice daily) has an antiandrogen effect. This should not be used in women who may get pregnant since it is teratogenic.
  ❑ Flutamide is a potent antiandrogen that is rarely used since it causes hepatotoxicity.
❑ 5-α reductase inhibitors:
  ❑ Finasteride (5 mg daily) is effective but is teratogenic. It blocks the conversion of testosterone to the more potent dihydrotestosterone.

Drugs used in managing amenorrhoea or oligomenorrhoea in PCOS include:
❑ OCP.
❑ Metformin (500 mg three times daily). This is frequently effective through improvements in insulin sensitivity and reduced SHBG and LH levels.

Infertility in PCOS is managed in a variety of ways including:
- ❑ Metformin.
- ❑ Clomiphene (25–150 mg days 5–9 of menstrual cycle). This inhibits the negative feedback from oestrogen, increasing FSH secretion. It is effective in two-thirds of patients. It can be used for up to six cycles.
- ❑ Low-dose gonadotrophin therapy.
- ❑ Laparoscopic ovarian diathermy or laser drilling.
- ❑ *In vitro* fertilization.

Women with PCOS are at increased risk of developing Type 2 diabetes and, therefore, cardiovascular disease. They should be monitored annually for cardiovascular risk including blood pressure, blood glucose, and lipid measurements.

Androgen-secreting tumours

Androgen-secreting tumours of the ovary or adrenal gland should be treated by surgical removal. Malignant tumours tend to be unresponsive to chemotherapy or radiotherapy. The 5-year survival rates are <30%.

REPRODUCTIVE HORMONE DEFICIENCIES

Premature ovarian failure (POF) and the menopause

Women with POF have an increased risk of osteoporosis and circulatory disease. They are also frequently symptomatic. It is therefore important that oestrogen replacement in the form of hormone replacement therapy (HRT) is instituted until menopause would have been anticipated (about 50 years). In women with an intact uterus, progesterone should be added since unopposed oestrogens increase the risk of endometrial carcinoma. This is usually given for half the menstrual cycle or as a daily low-dose preparation. HRT replacement is generally given in tablet form. Oestrogen is also available as a transdermal patch, gel, and subcutaneous implant (6 monthly).

For infertility, oocyte donation and *in vitro* fertilization is successful in one-third of patients. For hot flushes, megestrol acetate and clonidine may be useful agents in controlling symptoms in those women who cannot take HRT.

The risks and benefits of prescribing HRT in postmenopausal women are described in *Table 65*. A short course (<5 years) of HRT is generally recommended now for patients with distressing symptoms. There are a number of clear contraindications for its use:

- ❑ Breast and endometrial cancer.
- ❑ Active or at high risk for deep venous thrombosis.
- ❑ Active liver disease.
- ❑ Unexplained vaginal bleeding.
- ❑ Active liver disease.
- ❑ Dyslipidaemia with raised serum triglycerides.

Turner's syndrome

Women with Turner's syndrome should be given HRT and receive regular screening for complications. This should include the following investigations:
- ❑ Baseline renal ultrasound scan.
- ❑ Annual blood pressure.
- ❑ Annual lipid profile.
- ❑ Annual fasting blood glucose.
- ❑ Annual blood pressure.
- ❑ 3-yearly echocardiogram.
- ❑ 3-yearly bone densitometry.

Male hypogonadism

There is a number of reasons for treating the male with hypogonadism:
- ❑ To improve symptoms (libido, erectile dysfuction, virilization, well being, and mood).
- ❑ To improve body composition (increase muscle mass, reduce body fat).
- ❑ To improve fertility.
- ❑ To prevent osteoporosis.

With the exception of fertility, testosterone replacement will achieve these aims.

Table 65 Risks and benefits of prescribing HRT in postmenopausal women

Benefits
- ❑ Alleviation of symptoms
- ❑ Reduction in risk of osteoporosis
- ❑ Reduction in risk of Alzheimer's disease

Risks
- ❑ Potential increased risk of ischaemic heart disease
- ❑ Increased risk of breast cancer
- ❑ Side-effects (breast tenderness, mood changes, irregular vaginal bleeding)

Testosterone is, however, contraindicated in patients with prostate or breast cancer. It may worsen polycythaemia, sleep apnoea, and prostate enlargement. Other potential side-effects include mood changes, acne, gynaecomastia (especially in prepuberty), and hepatotoxicity. Testosterone can be given intramuscularly, typically as Sustanon 250 mg every 3 weeks in the adult. Recently, gel preparations (Testimgel and Testogel) have proved popular. Gels are administered once daily to the shoulder, upper arm, or abdomen, avoiding washing the area for several hours after application. Transdermal scrotal and nonscrotal patches have proved less popular. Nonscrotal patches are frequently associated with a skin rash. Testosterone implants, typically 400–600 mg 6-monthly, are preferred by some. Oral testosterone preparations are highly variable with most failing to achieve satisfactory serum levels of testosterone.

Monitoring of testosterone levels in addition to a prostate examination, prostate-specific antigen (PSA), full blood count, and liver and lipid profiles is recommended at least annually. Testosterone levels should be kept in the normal range (*Table 66*) with the aim of symptomatic improvement.

Table 66 Endocrine testing: normal ranges

Laboratory parameter	SI	Conventional
Adrenal steroids, plasma		
Aldosterone, supine, saline suppression	<240 pmol/l	<8.5 ng/dl
Aldosterone, upright, normal diet	140–560 pmol/l	5–20 ng/dl
Cortisol		
8 am	140–690 nmol/l	5–25 µg/dl
4 pm	80–330 nmol/l	3–12 µg/dl
Overnight dexamethasone suppression	<140 nmol/l	<5 µg/dl
Dehydroepiandrostenedione (DHEA)	7–31 nmol/l	2–9 µg/dl
Dehydroepiandrostenedione sulfate (DHEAS)	1.3–6.8 µmol/l	500–2500 ng/ml
11-Deoxycortisol	<30 nmol/l	< 1 µg/dl
17-Hydroxyprogesterone		
Women, follicular phase	0.6–3 nmol/l	0.2–1 µg/l
Women, luteal phase	1.5–10.6 nmol/l	0.5–3.5 µg/l
Men	1.8–9 nmol/l	0.6–3 µg/l
Adrenal steroids, urine		
Aldosterone	14–53 nmol/d	5–19 µg/d
Cortisol, free	55–276 nmol/d	20–100 µg/d
17-Hydroxycorticosteroids	5.4–27.6 µmol/d	2–10 mg/d
Adrenocorticotrophic hormone (ACTH), plasma 8 am	2–11 pmol/l	9–52 pg/ml
Angiotensin II, plasma	10–60 ng/l	10–60 pg/ml
Arginine vasopressin (AVP), plasma		
Random fluid intake	0–2.8 pmol/l	1–3 pg/ml
Dehydration 18–24 hr	5.5–13 pmol/l	4–14 pg/ml
Vitamin D		
1,25-Dihydroxycholecalciferol (1,25[OH]2D)	36–144 pmol/l	15–60 pg/ml
25-Hydroxycholecalciferol (25-OH-D)	20–100 nmol/l	8–40 ng/ml
Calcitonin, plasma		
Normal	<19 ng/l	<19 pg/ml
Medullary cancer	>100 ng/l	>100 pg/ml

Laboratory parameter	SI	Conventional
Calcium		
Ionized serum	1–1.4 mmol/l	4–5.6 mg/dl
Total serum	2.2–2.6 mmol/l	9–10.5 mg/dl
Catecholamines, urine		
Free	<590 nmol/d	<100 µg/d
Epinephrine	<275 nmol/d	<50 µg/d
Metanephrines	<7 µmol/d	<1.3 ng/d
Norepinephrine	89–473 nmol/d	15–89 µg/d
Vanillylmandelic acid (VMA)	<40 µmol/d	<8 mg/d
Chloride, serum	98–106 µmol/l	98–106 mEq/l
Gastrin, plasma	<120 ng/l	<120 pg/ml
Glucagon, plasma	50–100 ng/l	50–100 pg/ml
Glucose, plasma		
Overnight fast, normal	4.2–6.4 mmol/l	75–115 mg/dl
Overnight fast, diabetes mellitus	>7.0 mmol/l	>126 mg/dl
72-h fast, normal men	>2.8 mmol/l	>50 mg/dl
72-h fast, normal women	>2.2 mmol/l	>40 mg/dl
Glucose Tolerance Test, 2-h postprandial plasma glucose		
Normal	<7.8 mmol/l	<140 mg/dl
Impaired glucose tolerance	7.8–11.1 mmol/l	140–200 mg/dl
Diabetes mellitus	>11.1 mmol/l	>200 mg/dl
Gonadal steroids, plasma		
Androstenedione		
Women	3.5–7.0 nmol/l	1–2 ng/ml
Men	3.0–5.0 nmol/l	0.8–1.3 ng/ml
Dihydrotestosterone		
Women	0.17–1 nmol/l	0.05–3 ng/ml
Men	0.87–2.6 nmol/l	0.25–0.75 ng/ml
Oestradiol		
Women, basal	70–220 pmol/l	20–60 pg/ml
Women, ovulatory surge	>740 pmol/l	>200 pg/ml
Men	<180 pmol/l	<50 pg/ml
Progesterone		
Women, luteal phase	6–64 nmol/l	2–20 ng/ml
Women, follicular phase	<6 nmol/l	<2 ng/ml
Men	<6 nmol/l	<2 ng/ml
Testosterone		
Women	<3.5 nmol/l	<1 ng/ml
Men	10–35 nmol/l	3–10 ng/ml
Gonadotrophins, plasma		
Follicle stimulating hormone (FSH)		
Women, basal	1.4–9.6 IU/l	1.4–9.6 mIU/ml
Women, ovulatory surge	2.3–21 IU/l	2.3–21 mIU/ml
Women, postmenopausal	34–96 IU/l	34–96 mIU/ml
Men	0.9–15 IU/l	0.9–15 mIU/ml
Luteinizing hormone (LH)		
Women, basal	0.8–26 IU/l	0.8–26 mIU/ml

(Continued overleaf)

Laboratory parameter	SI	Conventional
Gonadotrophins, plasma, Luteinizing hormone (LH) (*continued*)		
Women, ovulatory surge	25–57 IU/l	25–57 mIU/ml
Women, postmenopausal	40–104 IU/l	40–104 mIU/ml
Men	1.3–13 IU/l	1.3–13 mIU/ml
Growth horone (GH), plasma		
After 100 g glucose orally	<2 µg/l	<2 ng/ml
After insulin-induced hypoglycaemia	>9 µg/l	>9 ng/ml
Insulin, plasma		
Fasting	35–145 pmol/l	5–20 uU/ml
During hypoglycaemia (plasma glucose)	<2.8 nmol/l, <50 mg/ml)	<35 pmol/l <5 uU/ml
Insulin C peptide	0.5–2 µg/l	0.5–2 pg/ml
Insulin-like growth factor-1 (IGF-1)		
Women	0.45–2.2 kU/l	0.45–2.2 U/ml
Men	0.34–1.9 kU/l	0.34–1.9 U/ml
Lactate, plasma	0.56–2.2 mmol/l	5–20 mg/dl
Magnesium, serum	0.8–1.3 mmol/l	1.8–3 mg/dl
Osmolality, plasma	285–295 mmol/kg	285–295 mOsmol/l
Oxytocin, plasma		
Random	1–4 pmol/l	1.25–5 ng/l
Women, ovulatory surge	4–8 pmol/l	5–10 ng/l
Parathyroid hormone (PTH), serum	10–65 ng/l	10–65 pg/ml
Phosphorus, inorganic, serum	1–1.5 mmol/l	3–4.5 mg/dl
Prolactin, serum		
Nonpregnant women and men	2–15 µg/l	2–15 ng/ml
Renin activity, plasma, normal sodium intake		
Supine	3.2 ± 1 µg/l/h	3.2 ± 1 ng/ml/h
Standing	9.3 ± 4.3 µg/l/h	9.3 ± 4.3 mg/ml/h
Sodium, serum	136–145 mmol/l	136–145 mEq/l
Thyroid Function Tests		
Free thyroxine estimate	9–26 pmol/l	0.7–2 ng/dl
Radioactive iodine, uptake 24 h	0.05–0.3%	5–30%
Reverse triiodothyronine (rT$_3$), serum	0.15–0.61 nmol/l	10–40 ng/dl
Thyroid stimulating hormone (TSH), serum	0.5–5 mU/l	0.5–5 µU/ml
Thyroxine (T$_4$), serum	64–154 nmol/l	5–12 µg/dl
Triiodothyronine (T$_3$), serum	1.1–2.9 nmol/l	70–190 µg/dl

CASE 12

A 24-year-old woman presents with a history of worsening hirsuitism, obesity (BMI 32), and oligomenorrhoea over a period of several years. On examination she is overweight with increased quantities of coarse dark hair on the chin, upper lip, breasts, and inner thighs. There is no clitoromegaly. Her voice is normal and she is not excessively muscular. A diagnosis of PCOS is suspected.

1 What investigation results would support the presumed diagnosis?
2 What commonly used management steps might help alleviate her symptoms?

Answers to Case 12 on page 158.

CASE 1 ANSWER

1 A fingerprick (capillary) blood glucose measurement. This should be followed by a laboratory plasma glucose to confirm the elevated result.
2 DKA. This is a classical presentation of newly diagnosed Type 1 diabetes.
3 In view of the patient's fluctuating conscious level, it is important to ensure that the patient's airway is patent. Immediate treatment consists of intravenous fluid replacement (normal saline infused quickly) to correct the dehydration and intravenous insulin (6–8 units per hour) to correct the hyperglycaemia. Arterial blood gases should be performed to assess for the severity of acidosis.

CASE 2 ANSWER

1 i. This gentleman has HONK.
  ii. He is likely to be profoundly dehydrated (>5 litres).
  iii. He certainly requires fluid replacement but the rate at which it is replaced should depend upon his clinical response to an initial fluid load. He is at high risk of developing pulmonary oedema and a CVP line may need to be inserted so that his fluid requirements can be more accurately monitored.
2 There is likely to be an underlying cause for his deterioration. Common precipitating causes for HONK are myocardial infarction, stroke, pneumonia, and urinary tract infection. He needs a chest X-ray, echocardiogram, urinalysis, blood and urine culture. In view of his unconsciousness, an urgent brain CT scan may be indicated.

CASE 3 ANSWER

1 This patient has sight threatening proliferative retinopathy.
2 He should be referred the same day to an experienced Ophthalmologist (via Eye Casualty if necessary) so that laser therapy can be commenced.

CASE 4 ANSWER

1 This lady has thyrotoxicosis secondary to autoimmune Graves' disease. She is clinically and biochemically hyperthyroid with raised free T4 and suppressed TSH, indicating primary hyperthyroidism. The presence of eye signs and a smooth diffusely-enlarged thyroid gland is suggestive of Graves' disease.

2 Antithyroid drug therapy is indicated. Typically, carbimazole 30–40 mg once daily or propylthiouracil 100 mg t.d.s. is a sensible starting regime. Propranolol 10–40 mg t.d.s. will ease the symptoms of palpitations and tremor.

CASE 5 ANSWER

1 This woman has primary hypothyroidism. This suspected diagnosis is confirmed on biochemical testing by a low free T4 and markedly elevated TSH level.
2 Thyroid replacement therapy should be commenced. In view of this woman's heart disease, levothyroxine should be initiated at low dose (25 µg once daily). This should be increased gradually by 25 µg every 4 weeks until thyroid function tests are in the normal range.

CASE 6 ANSWER

1 An initial screen to exclude diabetes mellitus, hypokalaemia, renal impairment, and hypercalcaemia should be performed. Tests should include urinalysis, fasting plasma glucose, urea and electrolytes, and calcium estimation.
2 This man has primary or tertiary hyperparathyroidism. He should undergo imaging of parathyroid tissue, probably with a combination of digital subtraction scanning (e.g. Sestamibi) and high-resolution ultrasound. Once a parathyroid adenoma is localized he should undergo definitive surgical parathyroidectomy.

CASE 7 ANSWER

1 This woman has had positive screening and diagnostic tests for Cushing's syndrome. The suppressed ACTH measurement indicates that the site of her cortisol secretion is her adrenal gland(s). The most likely cause is therefore a cortisol-secreting adenoma of the adrenal gland.
2 After localization of the tumour by imaging, e.g. CT scanning of the adrenal glands, the definitive treatment consists of surgical adrenalectomy. The patient may be pretreated with cortisol-suppressant therapy (e.g. metyrapone or ketonacozole) accompanied by supplementation with hydrocortisone.

CASE 8 ANSWER

1 He has probable Addison's disease and requires a short synacthen test to confirm the diagnosis. He may require other investigations to establish the cause. These include adrenal autoantibodies, CT imaging of the abdomen, and microbiological investigations if an infective condition involving his adrenal glands is considered likely.

2 He will require steroid replacement therapy, typically given as hydrocortisone 10 mg on waking, 5 mg at noon, and 5 mg late afternoon. Mineralocorticoid replacement should be given in the form of fludrocortisone (typically 0.1 mg daily).

CASE 9 ANSWER

1 Common symptoms include increased sweating, headaches, tiredness and lethargy, joint pains, and change in shoe/ring size.

2 Medical complications include hypertension, diabetes mellitus, ischaemic heart disease, cardiac failure, colonic carcinoma, carpal tunnel syndrome, visual field defects, and hypopituitarism.

CASE 10 ANSWER

1 A PRL-secreting macroadenoma of the pituitary gland (prolactinoma). The markedly elevated PRL indicates a PRL-secreting tumour. The visual field deficit indicates extension of the tumour to compress partially the optic chiasm.

2 This is likely to represent a nonsecreting macroadenoma of the pituitary gland. The mildly elevated PRL relates to compression of the pituitary stalk. Differential diagnoses include compression of the pituitary stalk and optic chiasm by another space-occupying lesion, e.g. craniopharyngioma or meningioma.

3 Prochlorperazine is a dopamine antagonist and will cause an elevation of serum PRL.

CASE 11 ANSWER

1 Hypopituitarism. This is suggested by the clinical history. The investigation results indicate secondary hypothyroidism and a reduced level of testosterone.

2 A serum cortisol should be checked urgently. If this man has panhypopituitarism then he will need urgent steroid replacement. He will almost certainly require MRI imaging of his pituitary gland.

3 If he is cortisol deficient then he should be commenced on hydrocortisone replacement therapy. After 1 week of hydrocortisone replacement, it would be safe and appropriate to commence oral thyroxine. He may subsequently require testosterone replacement therapy. This will depend upon investigations and management of his hypopituitarism.

CASE 12 ANSWER

1

❏ A raised serum LH/FSH ratio (LH concentration is frequently elevated in patients with PCOS).

❏ Low levels of SHBG. The elevated SHBG is secondary to hyperinsulinaemia and leads to elevated free, unbound circulating testosterone.

❏ Normal or marginally elevated serum testosterone. Other causes of hyperandrogenism, e.g. virilizing tumours, are associated with raised testosterone.

❏ Transvaginal pelvic ultrasound. Multiple ovarian follicular cysts and thickened ovarian stroma are frequently seen in women with PCOS.

2

❏ Weight loss. This will reduce insulin resistance and hyperandrogenaemia, helping to reduce obesity, hirsuitism, and restore a regular menstrual cycle.

❏ Local hair removal. Waxing and shaving can be effective short-term therapies for hirsuitism. Electrolysis and laser therapy offer more permanent solutions. Topical eflornithine (Vaniqa) applied twice daily is an effective licensed preparation for facial hirsuitism.

❏ Oestrogen supplementation. The OCP is effective since oestrogen reduces SHBG levels and, therefore, reduces free androgen concentrations, aiding hirsuitism, and inducing a regular withdrawal bleed.

❏ Antiandrogen therapy. Dianette, an OCP that contains 2 mg cyproterone acetate, is effective for cycle regulation and hirsuitism. Higher doses of cyproterone can be prescribed in combination with an OCP for hirsuitism. Spironolactone is a weak anti-androgen. Flutamide is a more potent antiandrogen.

❏ Insulin sensitizers. Metformin has been used with success for regulating the menstrual cycle and restoring fertility. It is not an effective therapy for hirsuitism.

❏ 5-α reductase inhibition. Finasteride, 5 mg daily, blocks the conversion of testosterone to the more potent dihydrotestosterone and is effective for hirsuitism. It is, however, teratogenic and should be avoided when pregnancy is a possibility.

Index

Shape

Karen Bryant-Mole

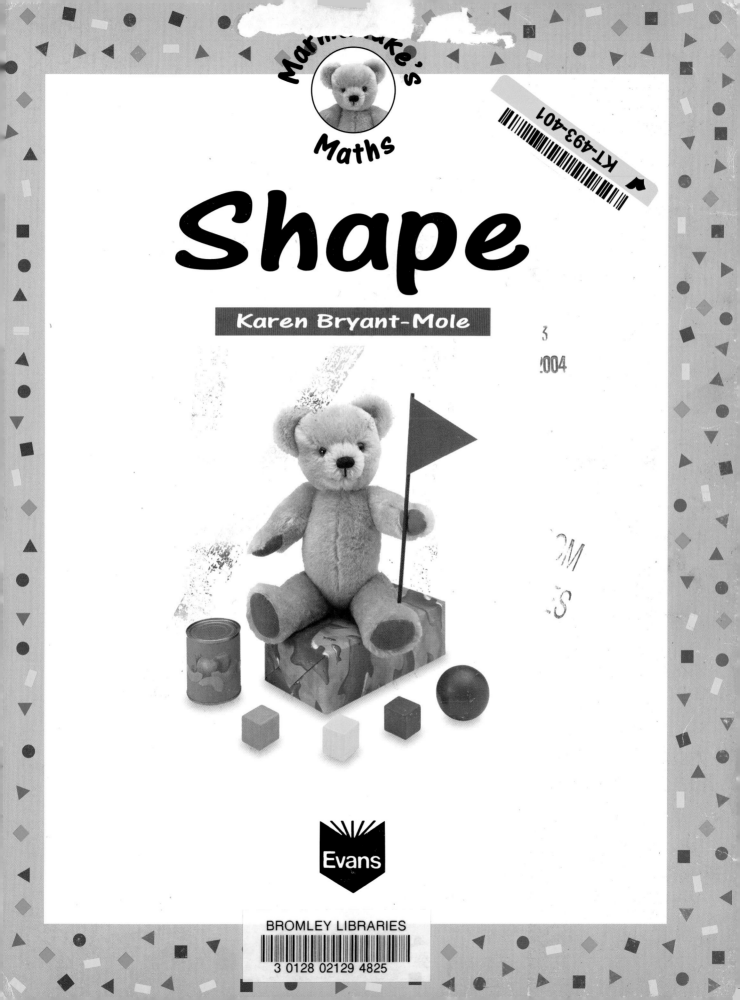

Evans

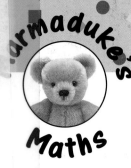

Pattern ● Shape ● Size
Sorting ● Where is Marmaduke?

Published by Evans Brothers Limited
2A Portman Mansions
Chiltern Street
London W1M 1LE

© BryantMole Books 1999

First published in 1999
First published in paperback 1999

Printed in Hong Kong by Wing King Tong Co Ltd

British Library Cataloguing in Publication Data

Bryant-Mole, Karen
  Shape. - (Marmaduke's Maths)
  1.Marmaduke (Fictitious character) - Juvenile literature
  2.Geometrical constructions - Juvenile literature
  3.Form perception - Juvenile literature
  I.Title
  516.1'5

  ISBN 0 237 52121 0

The name **Marmaduke** is a registered trade mark.

Created by Karen Bryant-Mole
Photographed by Zul Mukhida
Designed by Jean Wheeler
Teddy bear by Merrythought Ltd

About this book

Marmaduke the bear helps children to understand mathematical concepts by guiding them through the learning process in a fun, friendly way.

This book introduces children to the concept of shape. Children are introduced to the idea that there are two different types of shape, 2D and 3D, and are taught how individual shapes can be defined. Everyday examples help children to recognise these shapes.

You can use this book as a starting point for further work on shape. It is very important that shape words are used correctly. Objects that are described in 2D terms must be flat. Balls are not circles, they are spheres. Look out for shapes all around you. Kitchen cupboards are good places to find cubes, cuboids and cylinders. Watch out for road signs in the shape of circles, rectangles and triangles.

contents

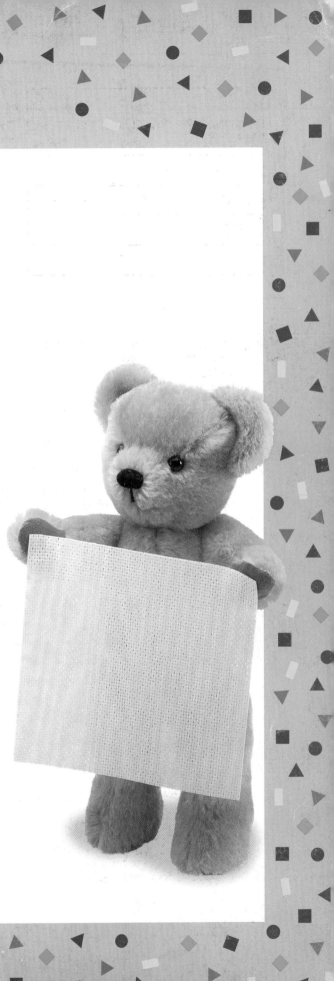

shapes

Marmaduke is cutting out some shapes
from coloured paper.

Paper is very thin.
All the shapes are flat.

Flat shapes are
sometimes called
2D shapes.

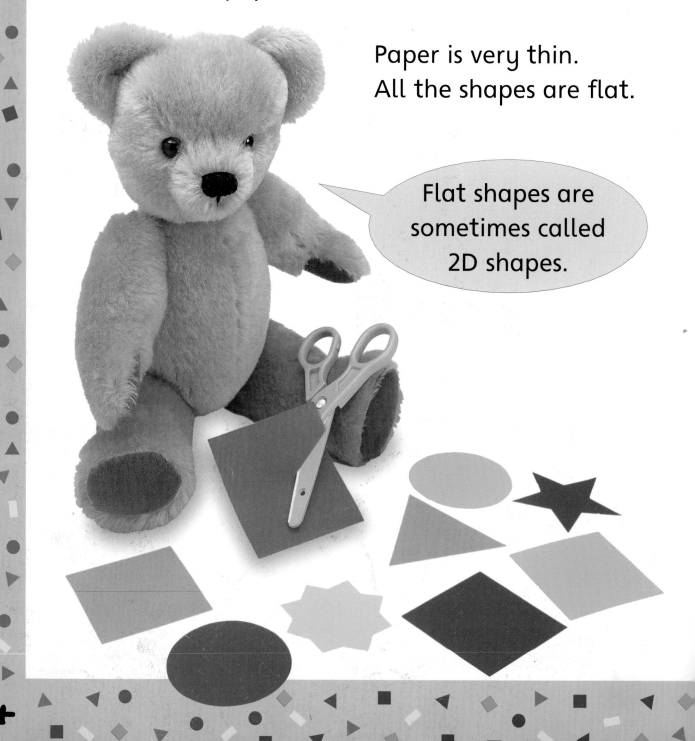

Marmaduke's bricks are not flat.
Shapes that are not flat are called solid shapes.

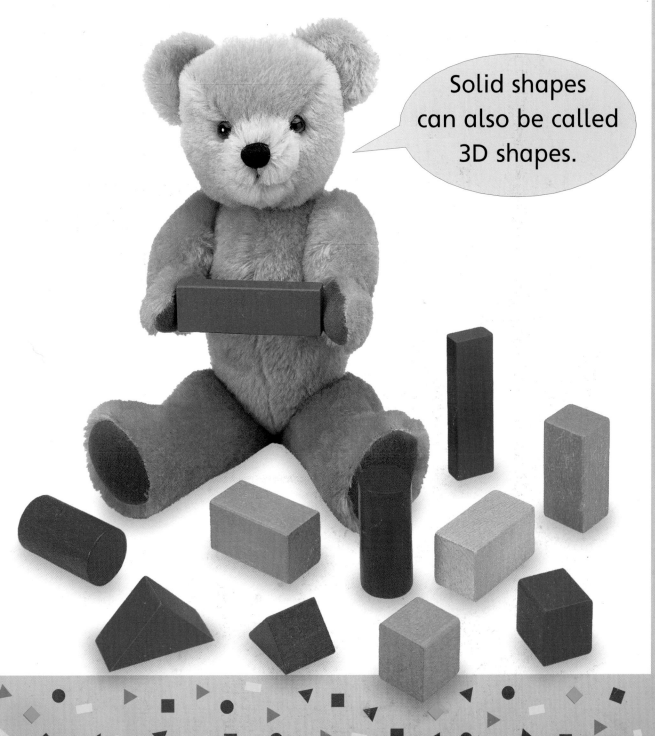

Solid shapes can also be called 3D shapes.

circle

Marmaduke is
wearing a big badge.

The shape of
my badge is called
a circle.

Circles are flat shapes.
They have no corners.
They have one curved side that
goes all the way round.

All of these things are circles.

some buttons

a biscuit

some coins

rectangle

Marmaduke has been sent a postcard.

The shape of this postcard is a rectangle.

Rectangles are flat shapes.
They have four corners and four straight sides.

Here are some more rectangles.

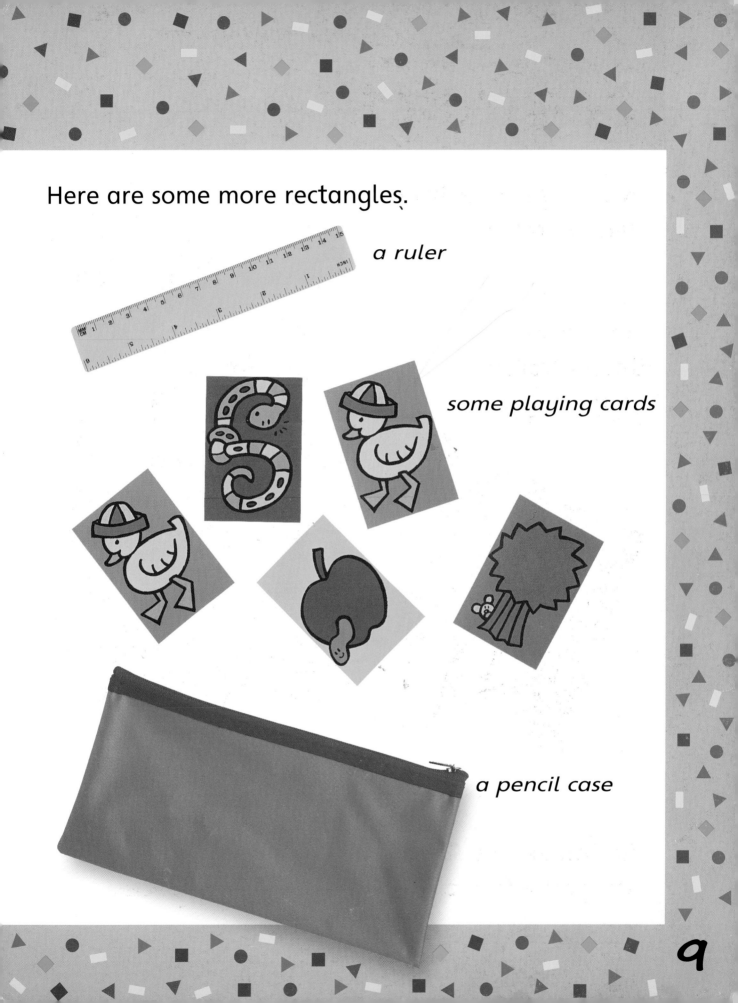

a ruler

some playing cards

a pencil case

square

Marmaduke is going to wash some dishes.
He is holding a dishcloth.

The shape of my dishcloth is a square.

Squares are special rectangles.
All the sides are the same length.

Here are some more squares that Marmaduke found around his home.

a flannel

a duster

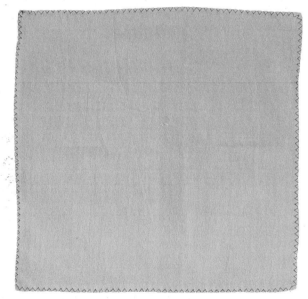

a paper serviette

triangle

Marmaduke is waving a flag.

The shape of this flag is a triangle.

Triangles are flat shapes. They have three straight sides and three corners.

These shapes are all triangles but
they all look very different.
Count the sides and the corners.

sphere

Marmaduke is holding a blue ball.

The shape of this ball is a sphere.

Spheres are solid shapes.
They are perfectly round.
Spheres roll very easily.

Here are some more balls.
They are all spheres but
they are different sizes.

cylinder

Marmaduke has been shopping.
He bought a tin of fruit.

The shape of
this tin is called
a cylinder.

Cylinders are solid shapes.
They are like tubes with closed ends.

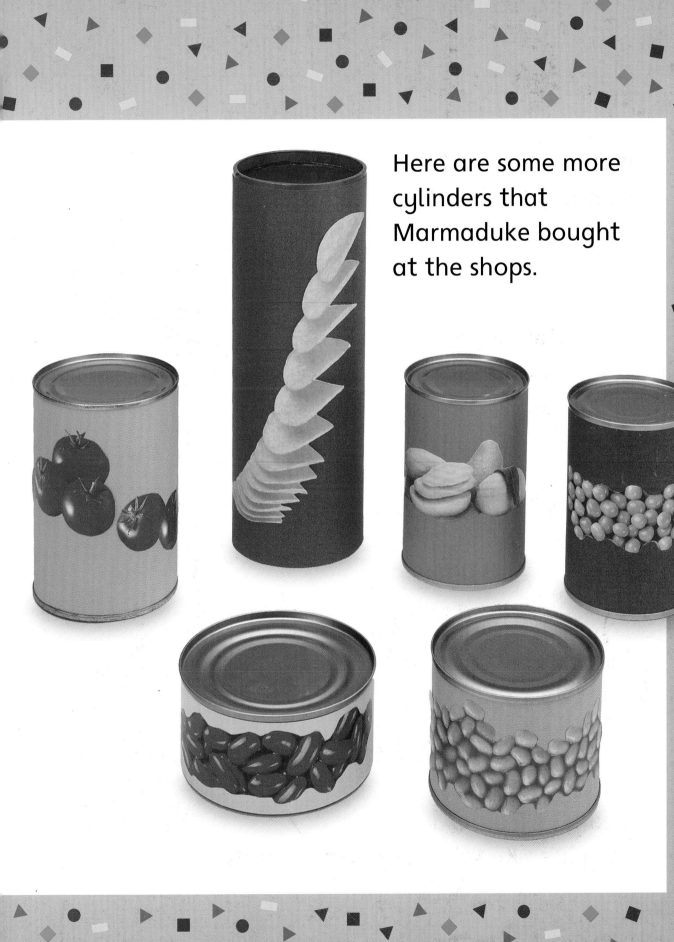

Here are some more cylinders that Marmaduke bought at the shops.

cuboid

It is Marmaduke's birthday.
He has been given
a present.

The shape of
this present is called
a cuboid.

Cuboids are solid shapes.
Some sides of a cuboid are longer than others.

Here are some
more presents.
They are
all cuboids.

Which is which?

Marmaduke is trying to remember the names of all the shapes.

Can you help me?

If you cannot remember, look back
through the book.
Marmaduke has already shown you
each of these objects.

glossary

dice cubes with different numbers of dots on their sides, thrown in board games

flannel sometimes called a face cloth

playing cards cards used to play card games, such as Snap and Pairs

ruler an object used to measure how long things are

serviette an object used to wipe your mouth or fingers when you are eating a meal

tissues paper handkerchiefs that are thrown away after they have been used

index